SUNFOOD Cuisine

SUNFOOD Cuisine

FREDERIC PATENAUDE

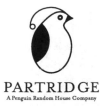

PARTRIDGE
A Penguin Random House Company

To order additional copies of this book, contact
Partridge India
000 800 10062 62
www.partridgepublishing.com/india
orders.india@partridgepublishing.com

CONTENTS

DEDICATION

The author would also like to thank all the people who have contributed to the original version of this book (first published as "The Sunfood Cuisine", including the following:

Andrew Ethan Durham—For testing all my recipes, and being my friend.

Annie Jubb—For the inspiration.

Barbara Stead—For letting me stay at the Ranch.

Craig Lowellen "Emerald Spider"—For all I have learned from you during the WBF training, and after.

Dr. David Jubb—For all the teachings.

David Norman—For the pictures, and all the amazing help.

David Wolfe—For printing and publishing the first edition of this book.

Dianne Onstad—For reading, re-reading, editing and getting this book ready for print.

Durian—For helping without asking anything in return.

Fred Silverbear—For patiently testing all my recipes back in January 2000!

Jeremy Safron—For the raw chef skills.

John McCabe—For all the help, amazing insights, and sparkling ideas.

Liz—For testing some of the recipes, and for the support.

Louiselle—Merci pour m'avoir mis au monde.

Marianne Moineau—Pour avoir toujours cru en ce projet, et en moi.

Michael McCarthy—For the encouragement, insights, constant support, and for the raw yoga!

Morten Blakestone—For providing a roof at a time when I had little money, and nowhere to go.

Olivier Magnan—Pour les enseignements!

Raven Pelan—For encouraging me to finish this book. "You need to finish your book Fred, I need it!"

Real Patenaude—Pour étre mon pére préféré!

Sara Honeycutt—For her inspiring conceptual art that graces the cover and pages of this book.

Sébastien Patenaude—Pour étre mon frére, mon ami, et mon fan.

Sequoia Neptune—For the yoga!

Stephen Arlin—For the time at NFL, the laughs, and all the help.

Suzie Bohannon—For the raw chef skills.

INTRODUCTION

"The sun is the source of all life on this planet." This is a powerful concept we all know and, to some degree, one that is part of all mythologies. For as long as humans have existed, they have been aware of the power of the sun. It is what makes plants grow and without it, no life would be possible on this planet. When the sun shines, everyone feels better, for the light of the sun is indispensable in keeping our bodies and spirits alive and alight.

Raw foods are plant-based foods that contain the life-force of the sun. Raw foods are the beautiful fruits, vegetables and nuts that have been grown in the sun, without the use of chemical fertilizers and pesticides. They carry within them all the radiant life-giving energy of the sun. They are alive because they have not been prepared using fire, heating, or cooking. Foods that have been cooked and denatured no longer carry that life-force.

Throughout this book you will learn a completely different approach to making foods. Instead of thinking in terms of frying, boiling, and roasting, you will be learning how to combine the intense flavors of fruits, vegetables, nuts, herbs and spices, to create tasty and healthy meals.

It is wonderful when, after a meal, you no longer need to scrub the grease off of your pots and pans. In fact, what the cooked foods do to your pots and pans is a testament to what they do in your body. The greasy and starchy foods often ferment inside of you, sticking to the walls of your intestines and clogging your system. On the other hand, clean foods leave clean dishes. And they leave you clean on the inside!

Eating an abundance of raw fruits and vegetables is one of the single most important things you can do to improve your health, your life, and your appearance. You will learn in this book about some of the marvelous properties of raw fruits and vegetables which, I am sure, will encourage you to include a large portion of these foods in your diet.

The recipes in this book are tasty and easy to prepare. To prepare them, you will only need a few basic pieces of kitchen equipment. But if all you have is a knife, a cutting board and a bowl, you will still be able to prepare most of the recipes.

Thank you for reading this book. It has been a pleasure to write, and it is an even greater pleasure to see people benefiting from it. I have put all of the love I could into the creation of the recipes, and if you put as much love into their preparation, you will be eating the most alive meals on the planet.

Frédéric Patenaude
April, 2003

NOTE: This book constitute an excerpt of the author's first book "The Sunfood Cuisine", first published in 2001. Because his research has evolved over the years, some of the ideas in this book may be in slight conflict with some of his newer research. However, these are for details and the basic philosophy stays the same. We hope that the reader will get great value from the content of this book, and will understand that the author's thoughts have been further defined in his next books.

Chapter 1
WHY RAW FOODS?

Many people throughout the world want to move away from their traditional diets of processed grains and animal products and towards a healthier diet. Research shows that the consumption of raw fruits and vegetables is one of the basic keys to good health. Many people know that raw fruits and vegetables are healthy foods and strive to eat them everyday. However, few realize that raw fruits and vegetables are so important that they should be your primary foods. This book will help you move away from the typical cooked, denatured and processed foods, and enter into the realm of raw and living foods—which I refer to as "Sunfoods."

There are many reasons why you should be eating mostly raw and living foods. Most of these reasons come from scientific research, and some of them from common sense—as well as the personal experience of millions of people throughout the world who have experienced the benefits of eating raw fruits and vegetables as the base of their diet.

IT MAKES SENSE

First, eating raw foods makes sense. Think about it. All creatures living on this planet thrive on a natural diet of raw plant foods. Humans are the only creatures cooking their food. Many have seen this as a great achievement, following the old belief that raw foods are hard to digest, and that cooking somehow improves their digestibility. Many scientists attribute all the greatest accomplishments of humanity to cooking and agriculture. But if this were true, then why are humans the sickest creatures on the planet? We are not thriving like wild animals are. Wild animals, living on raw foods, have an amazing vitality that enables them to survive the harshest living conditions. Could you imagine what would happen if a tribe of wild wolves started feeding on donuts and cooked meat? Do you think they would continue to thrive? Far from it. No creature can thrive on devitalized foods, and humans are no exception.

Eating raw foods makes sense because we are naturally attracted to these foods. Imagine for a second that you have been left on a desert island with no tools or technology. Now it's time to eat. What do you do? What are you naturally inclined to do? Start chasing a wild animal, catch it with your bare hands, and eat it alive? Find a cow and hope to be able to steal its milk? Graze? Catch a fish and eat it raw? Or maybe pick fruits and berries from the bushes and trees? Which option is the most appealing? I bet that the fruit option is. Why? Because this is what you are naturally attracted to. Humans are meant to eat raw fruits and vegetables—this is our natural diet.

Harvey Diamond, author of the wonderful book **Fit for Life**, which inspired so many people to eat their fruits and vegetables, used to say: "Give a baby a banana and a live rabbit. I can bet you my car that every single time the baby will eat the banana and play with the rabbit." The contrary would be quite a disturbing sight. Why do we feel it should be that way? Because this is how humans are meant to live.

Human babies have purer instincts than human adults, and are attracted to fruit. Why is it that many of the most popular foods made for children and babies are "fruit flavored," or shaped like fruit? Babies and children are naturally attracted to fruit, especially tropical fruits such as mangos and papayas. Children have to learn to enjoy the taste of meat and potatoes, but they naturally enjoy the taste of mangos, bananas, and papayas.

Eating raw fruits and vegetables makes sense because this is what we are supposed to eat. As you start eating more of these foods, you will likely realize that *this is the most natural and normal way to eat and live.*

COOKING DESTROYS
THE PATTERNS OF NATURE

Nature forms everything in patterns. There are patterns within the roots, trunks, stems, and branches of trees and plants. Patterns are also in the forms and colors of the leaves, flowers, fruits, and vegetables. On a smaller scale, there are patterns in the way the cells of the plants are arranged, and within the cells there are patterns in the DNA, and in the molecules. Nature also creates patterns in animals and humans. There are basic symmetrical patterns in the way the feet, legs, arms, and hands are formed. And there is symmetry in the features of the torso, face, and internal organs. The patterns formed by nature are seen throughout the body, including in the cells, DNA, and molecules.

What the act of cooking does is destroy what Nature has formed on a molecular level. Those who eat a raw-vegan diet are eating food the way Nature created it, with all of its nutrients and intricate molecular patterns

3

undamaged by heat. They are putting natural patterns into their body, which the body uses to create itself on a molecular level, and in a pattern that only Nature can create. Those who eat a cooked diet, whether it be a vegan, vegetarian or carnivorous diet, are putting into their mouths food which is no longer what Nature created, but that which is unnatural. Because of this, the cooked food eaters are likely to experience health conditions that are not seen in those who follow a natural, well-rounded, raw-vegan diet.

Science has shown over and over again that those who eat an unhealthy diet lacking in fresh fruits and vegetables are not as healthy as those who do. Those who eat certain types of cooked and unnatural foods experience certain types of health problems. Those who eat a lot of meat and animal products are likely to experience heart problems, and certain types of cancers. Those who eat diets lacking in certain nutrients are likely to experience certain health problems related to inadequate nutrition. But those who eat a well-rounded raw-vegan diet are much less likely to experience the health problems that are seen in the populations of people who follow cooked-food diets. Also, those who follow cooked-food diets are more likely to lack certain nutrients. This is because cooking destroys many nutrients. Eating raw-vegan foods provides better nutrition because the nutrients, including vitamins, minerals, amino acids, enzymes, and trace elements have not been destroyed or harmed by cooking.

WATER-RICH FOODS

Water is a critically important factor for good health. Many people understand the importance of drinking enough water, but few are able to live up to the recommendations given by doctors, which is to drink 8 to 10 large glasses of water every day.

Drinking plenty of water is important for many reasons. One is because water is largely what we are composed of, and it is constantly evaporating through our skin. Water is Nature's preferred solvent, and is used by the body to flush out toxins produced by the cells. If you do not take in enough water, you will experience symptoms associated with intoxication, such as headaches and constipation. Water is needed for the transportation of certain water-soluble nutrients. Also, the good bacteria that live in the intestines need water to survive.

One problem that most people have is that their food is largely devoid of living water. Everything you eat has to be turned into a liquid before your body can assimilate the nutrients within it. When you put a piece of bread into your mouth, your body has to use an incredible amount of energy to break it down, and rarely succeeds entirely in doing so. But when you eat a piece of fruit, such as a papaya which is mostly water, your body digests it with ease.

Water-rich foods are important because they keep the body clean. They are digested quickly, and the water in them helps to flush toxins out of the system. If you do not eat many water-rich foods, you will have to drink a lot of water to compensate. But the water that most people drink is quite toxic. Water coming out of a tap, and even some bottled water, is polluted with heavy metals and inorganic minerals. Also, water kept in plastic bottles contains gasses that leach out of the plastic.

The best and highest quality water can be found in fresh, organically grown fruits and vegetables. The water found in fruits and vegetables is pure because the plant itself through its roots has filtered it. There is no other source of water that matches the quality of water found in organically grown and wild plants.

Your body will function more regularly in the elimination department when fueled with the high-quality water found in organically grown fruits and vegetables. Cooked and dead foods have a tendency to clog the body. Raw fruits and vegetables do the opposite, and keep your system clean and running smoothly.

TOXINS IN COOKED FOOD

Cooked foods are the product of complex chemical reactions that even science has a difficult time understanding. Think about it: with a few basic pieces of equipment—a stove and a few pots and pans—you can radically transform your food, play with it, and transform its chemical composition on a molecular level. Think about the difference between a raw potato, and a potato after it has been baked. What a metamorphosis! And all of this you could not have achieved without this little magical feat you performed using the flames of your stove. But what is it that really goes on behind the scenes when we cook our foods? What is it that happens at the molecular level that can turn this raw potato into the food we know as a "baked potato?"

Cooking has always been considered an "art." Every possible way of transforming food has been permitted, as long as it was successful in creating something pleasing to the palate. This so-called art had the benefit of being able to use the rich, natural world to operate its marvels. It is possible, using the molecules contained in foods and transforming them using fire, to create countless new molecules that were not naturally present in the original foods. These new molecules are the true offspring of cooking, and their possible impact on human health is quite scary. Science is just starting to analyze these new creations of the cooking art, and because of the gigantic number of chemicals created by heat, there is no end in sight.

Rarely are chefs interested in the complexities of science, and it might scare them to think of their art as cold science. But the amazing laws of science only ask us to admit that our Universe is composed of molecules, which are in themselves composed of atoms. Living things are made up of patterns of cells, which are made up of patterns of molecules. Most of us have known this since grade school. We also know that atoms are linked together by chemical reactions that are stronger or weaker according to their type: between the atoms of a same molecule, the forces are generally strong, but between two different neighboring molecules the forces of attraction are weaken.

Often when we heat something, we break only the forces playing against the neighboring molecules. Turning water into ice is an example of stacking water molecules. When we heat ice, the energy that we bring suffices to break the links between the water molecules, and thus creates a liquid where the molecules, although forming a coherent mass, are moving from one another. However, in the liquid form, the molecules are not transformed, as the molecules of water are identical to the molecules of ice. Then again, when we heat water over 212 degrees (100 Celsius), it evaporates, because the heat that has been added is enough to break the forces of cohesion between the water molecules. Yet within each molecule the atom of oxygen is still linked to two atoms of hydrogen. This type of transformation is physical in its nature and not chemical: the water molecule stays a water molecule.

But, what the average chef does not know is that chemical reactions occur during the cooking process. This is because molecules in foods are being disassociated, rearranged, and new molecules are being created.

Here is what Guy Claude Burger wrote about one of the scientists working with the chemical changes in cooked foods (from **Manger Vrai**):

"In 1916, an American chemical engineer by the name of Maillard decided to isolate substances that give cooked foods their distinctive flavors, such as the tastes of bread, chocolate, and coffee. After having singled them out, he hoped, no doubt, to produce them artificially in order to add them to industrial foods and enhance the appeal that they could have to the consumer's taste buds. So, in order to complete his scheme, he had to determine the exact structure of these new molecules. He quickly found that these molecules resulted from very complex, haphazard chemical reactions between sugars and proteins, and one could produce them quite easily by heating any food even to moderate temperatures.

It is not possible to see with the naked eye what happens in a saucepan on the molecular level. When a chemist combines two substances in a test tube, and subsequently heats the compound over a Bunsen burner, it boils, clouds, changes color, or explodes accordingly. In each case, a new compound has been produced. Heat causes the molecules involved to collide, and repeated collision causes deviant bonding in order for new molecules, and hence a new substance, to form. The same goes for cooking, except that myriad molecules are brought together instead of just two.

In an ordinary baked potato, there are already 450 by-products of every description. They have even been named 'new chemical composites.' So far, around 50 such substances were studied and turned out to be either peroxiding, anti- oxidizing, or toxic, and possibly even mutagenic, meaning that they are liable to wreck cell nuclei and set up cancer. What was ascertained for broiled potatoes, which involves a fairly straightforward preparation, becomes much more serious with more sophisticated cookery. Sliced potatoes baked with cheese is a case in point. Heating releases an awesome array of chemical reactions—450 substances in potatoes, and probably many more in cheese, which is a highly intricate biochemical complex. Not only will those unwanted molecules stack up their effects, but, moreover, they will combine among themselves in every possible way—meaning that tens of thousands of abnormal substances will spring out of a cooked dish calling for mere potatoes and cheese. Just think of elaborate recipes where one clocks up endless chains of sundry ingredients jumbled together helter-skelter."

It seems that shortly after Maillard discovered these molecules—that have since been termed "Maillard's molecules"—he tried to prove that they had no adverse effect on human health. Some experiments quickly showed that he was wrong, and all his work was swept under the rug—until 1982, when some of his research appeared in scientific journals. Scientists are now beginning to see the connection between the introduction of these molecules into human bodies and common health problems.

From *Pyrolysis and Risks of Toxicity* by Professor R. Derache in "Cahiers de nutrition et de diztique" (Diet and nutrition Journal), 1982, p. 39:

"As far back as 1916, Maillard proved that the brown pigments and polymers that occur in pyrolysis (chemical breakdown by heat alone) . . . , are yielded after prior reaction of an amino acid group with the carbonyl group of sugars.

Though apparently simple, this reaction is, in fact, highly complex, itinerating in a spate of successive reactions and forming melanoidins, which are brown pigments that impart a typical color to whatever part of a food has endured higher temperatures.

The number of substances generated as a result is most impressive, yielding endless chains of new molecules: ketones, esters, aldehydes, ethers, volatile alcohols, and non-volatile heterocycles, etc. These innumerable substances coalesce into a complex compound, and are endowed with differing biological and chemical attributes: they are toxic, aromatic, peroxiding, anti-oxidizing, and possibly mutagenic and carcinogenic (DNA fractures can be oncogenic), or even antimutagenic and anti-carcinogenic. This to say that heating causes widespread disruption in the natural order of molecules."

The research backing this article evidenced over 50 pyrolytic substances in broiled potatoes alone, most of which originated from pyroseines and thiazole. However, Derache also states that "there remain, all in all, some 400 by-products to identify."

The brown color that chefs try to obtain while sautéing foods in oil is a color created through the Maillard reaction. The reaction occurs when high temperatures are reached by the fat content in food. It occurs less often when we boil foods because temperatures there are limited to the temperature of boiling water (212 degrees Fahrenheit, or 100 degrees Celsius).

The Maillard reaction is one type of possible reaction occurring during common food preparation, but not the only one. Cooked foods are the product of chemical reactions, and most transformations operated by the culinary art are chemical in their nature. When meat darkens on the surface as it is cooked, this is the result of a chemical reaction; when brown rice softens when boiled, this is also a chemical reaction. Unlike water, the molecules in food are extremely complex and fragile, leaving places for a huge amount of new chemistry in the cooking pan.

Cooking food is more than just one reaction—it is a mass of innumerable complex reactions that we simplify using the classifications of biochemists: carbohydrates, fats, proteins, water and minerals. The products of these reactions are innumerable, and still mostly unknown.

There are multiple reasons to believe that new molecules created during the process of cooking enter the blood stream without being properly digested, since there are no enzymes adapted for their digestion. These molecules would then accumulate in all parts of the body to create any number of conditions that we commonly refer to as diseases.

Many researchers think that there is no reason for the body to be adapted to the new molecules created in the process of cooking due to their huge quantities and complexity, and the fact that they have entered human bodies only in the past 10,000 years of human history.

The Maillard reaction works simultaneously upon thousands of compounds with innumerable combinations. When we cook food, we create molecules of unknown consequence to human health. So it is not hard to see how some of these molecules, in minimal concentration, could be at the origin of many serious health problems.

VITAMINS, MINERALS AND ANTIOXIDANTS

Raw fruits and vegetables are filled with vitamins and minerals which cooked and denatured foods lack because many nutrients are damaged and destroyed during the cooking process.

It is quite obvious that cooking destroys the nutritional quality of food since heating is a destructive process in itself. When you apply fire to something, it becomes less than it was. When you apply fire to your food, it becomes less than it was. You cannot "add" to your food by cooking it. You can only "subtract" from it, or alter it. When you fry vegetables, do they become more or less than they were before? They become less. They lose some of their nutritional value because fire destroys and does not create. Try putting your finger into the boiling water next time you make pasta (not for too long!), and you will realize what I mean by this "destructive process" we refer to as "cooking."

Your finger will get burned if you leave it in the boiling water. Your food is also burned and damaged when you boil or heat it in any way . . . cooking kills your food, metaphorically speaking!

Many nutrients are lost during the cooking process. Some foods that most people eat nearly every day are devoid of nutrients. For example, white bread does not contain any intrinsic vitamins. The only vitamins that it may contain are artificial vitamins that have been added to the bread. Canned goods also hardly contain any vitamins. Sailors travelling the oceans who lived on canned and other preserved foods eventually suffered from a serious disease caused by a vitamin deficiency—scurvy. It was soon discovered that adding citrus fruits to the diet of sailors could prevent scurvy.

When the body ingests a food that is deficient in vitamins and other important nutrients, not even speaking of enzymes, it has to provide its own supply of vitamins and nutrients in order to break it down. When the food takes more from the body than it gives in return you have a negative equation. For example, you may be eating something that has iron in it, but in order for your body to assimilate the iron, it needs some vitamins. If the vitamins are not present in the foods, your body will have to supply its own vitamins to absorb the minerals present in the foods. Better to eat foods that have all of their vitamin and mineral content intact. When you eat a variety of raw fruits and vegetables, you are sure to get the whole complement of vitamins and minerals that you need. Most fruits and vegetables are packed with vitamins and minerals that work in conjunction with each other. For example, papayas have a good supply of both calcium and vitamin C. The body needs vitamin C to assimilate calcium.

Eating a diet based on raw fruits and vegetables, and low in cooked and processed foods, maximizes the absorption of nutrients. Remember that many nutrients, and combinations of them that play an important role in your health, probably have not been discovered yet. Some of the most interesting discoveries about food and health have occurred in recent years as scientists have identified important elements in common fruits and vegetables that play a part in the prevention of certain diseases, such as heart disease and cancers. When we eat processed foods we eat foods that have less nutritional value and fewer of the important factors that have yet to be discovered. The only way to play it safe is to base your diet on raw fruits and vegetables, because we know that these foods have full nutrition, and unless they are processed and cooked, they can provide the body with the important nutrients that are needed.

INTESTINAL CLOGGING AND CONSTIPATION

A problem with the typical cooked-food diet is that it eventually leads to intestinal clogging, constipation, and it also clogs and constipates the entire body on a cellular level. The numerous chemicals that are created during the cooking process leave a residue throughout the body which slows the elimination of waste from the cells, each of which use energy and has its own system of elimination.

You probably understand the importance of good elimination. If your intestines do not function properly, nothing else will. Many have said that constipation is at the base of many diseases, and observation seems to support this concept in many ways. If the intestines become clogged, all the waste products from the rest of the organs and cells of the body also back up.

Ideally your intestinal transit time should be less than 20 hours. This means that after you eat something, it should come out the other end in less than 20 hours. This way the food does not putrefy in the intestines and poison the whole body. But on a typical diet rich in meat and grain products, food stays in the intestines for longer than a day, sometimes days at a time. Many people on cooked-food diets have problems with regularity, and have to resort to drugs in order to experience a bowel movement on a daily basis.

If you want to know how long it takes for your body to process your food, add whole sesame seeds to one of your meals. Whole sesame seeds will not be digested, and will be eliminated intact. This will let you know how long it takes your body to eliminate. If your typical elimination time is more than 20 hours, you should seriously consider improving your diet.

One of the first things that should be eliminated from your diet is animal products, especially meat. Meat has a tendency to remain an especially long time in the intestines of humans and putrefy. Humans simply do not have the capacity to digest meat properly.

True carnivores have very short intestines that allow them to rapidly process and eliminate the meat they eat. But within our human bodies, with our much longer intestines, meat putrefies as it makes its way through the system, and this produces many toxins. The foods we are meant to eat (fruits and vegetables) do not tend to putrefy. Since they are mostly water, they can benefit from a longer transit time in the intestines in order for the body to absorb maximum nutrition from them.

Grain products such as bread also have a tendency to ferment in the digestive tract and clog the system. Bread is made out of flour and water. What else is made out of flour and water? Glue! The sticky paste that comes from bread and flour products acts like glue in your body, and clogs your system.

Fruits and vegetables are clean foods that leave you clean inside. They are easy to digest, and easy to eliminate. Once they form the major part of your diet, rather than meat and grain products, you will finally experience proper digestion and elimination.

DIRTY ARTERIES

Your intestines are not the only part of your body that gets obstructed on a typical cooked food diet. Your arteries also get clogged. At the time of this writing, heart-related disease remains the most prevalent cause of death in North America and Europe. Clogged arteries are killing people on these continents by the millions every year.

All the research on heart disease seems to point to the following: diet is strongly linked to heart disease, and the best way to improve your diet is to reduce your intake of meat and other saturated fat-containing foods, while increasing your consumption of fresh fruits and vegetables.

It has been demonstrated that saturated fat triggers the bad cholesterol in your body to rise, which leads to clogged arteries and eventually heart disease. But not all types of fat are bad for you. The fat found in avocados, olives, flax seeds, hemp seeds, and other nuts and seeds have been shown to reduce the amount of bad cholesterol. This is one of the reasons why people living in the Mediterranean regions, while eating a diet high in fat, have a low incidence of heart disease compared to

Americans. This is because most of the fat they eat comes from cold-pressed olive oil, and other plant sources.

Fat found in meat, on the other hand, has been shown to cause heart disease and clogged arteries. Many people experience a significant reduction in their cholesterol level just by becoming vegetarian. Nations that are the heaviest meat eaters, such as United States and Canada, have the highest incidence of heart disease. Researchers have also found that certain components in raw fruits and vegetables help to keep the arteries clean; thus, raw plant foods not only do not cause heart disease in the first place, but can help reverse the condition by cleaning the arteries.

CANCER

Another common cause of pain and death in industrialized societies is cancer. About one quarter of the population in North America is affected by cancer at some point or another, and many die from it. Although scientists have promised many cures since U.S. President Richard Nixon declared a "war on cancer" over thirty years ago, none of the research has led anywhere. More people are dying of cancer every year in the U.S. than died of it thirty years ago. It has been found that cancer is strongly related to diet and lifestyle. Everyone knows that smoking causes lung cancer, but few are willing to admit that steak causes colon cancer, even though there is enough research to prove it.

On the other hand, it is in raw fruits and vegetables that we find the highest concentration of cancer-fighting components, such as antioxidants like vitamin C. Many studies have shown that diets that include plenty of raw fruits and vegetables are associated with a lower risk of cancer.

By eating a diet consisting of raw plant foods, you are lowering your chances of getting cancer in two ways. First, you are not ingesting most of the food substances that cause it; and second, you are eating the foods that help to prevent it.

BIOLOGICAL ADAPTATION

I have a belief, and I cannot tell you if it is true. I just know it to be true. This belief tells me that Nature did not make a mistake when She created life on this planet. Nature provided food for all of Her creatures, and I believe that She provided food for us too. All the creatures on this planet seem to find foods in their environment without needing to transform it in any way. All creatures on this planet have a natural diet, which they live on, and I believe that humans are no exception. I believe that we can find everything we need to eat right from the trees and the plants, without needing to transform or alter it in any way. When we cook foods because we think cooking makes them more digestible, it is like saying that Nature made a mistake when presenting us with the foods in their natural state. Wouldn't it make more sense if we ate food in the form Nature created it for us, and not feel compelled to transform it from its natural state?

Our natural foods are raw fruits and vegetables. These are the foods we are attracted to in their natural state. We enjoy eating fruits on their own, munching on lettuce and celery, and also snacking on raw nuts and seeds. But who likes to shove raw meat down their throat, or take a handful of raw grains and eat them? Nobody does (or almost nobody), because these foods do not taste great in their natural state. We have to cook them in order to enjoy them. And I believe that Nature gave us the senses of taste and smell so we could determine what is good to eat and what is not. Ideally, I would say that if it does not taste good in its raw, natural state, then maybe you should not be eating it.

Do not take my word for everything that I have said in this chapter. Try it for yourself I cannot convince you of anything. I did not write this book to sell you a belief. Your own intuition and judgement will tell you what is right for you, which may not be the same as what is right for me, or for your neighbor. But let me ask you to do something: just try it! Try living on nothing but raw fruits and vegetables, eating them in abundance, and see what happens to both your physical and mental states. Eat at least 80% raw fruits and vegetables, using the recipes in the book "**Easy Gourmet Raw Food Cuisine**", for the next two weeks and see how you feel. Then go back to eating less than 10% raw fruits and vegetables, and compare the difference. Anyone can do something for two weeks, especially if there is a possibility it may change his or her life in a great way.

You will inevitably find, when you eat more fruits and vegetables, you feel better. And that the heavy meals of meat, milk, and cooked starches sap your energy and vitality.

This is the power of Sunfood: fruits and vegetables contain vitality from the sun. When you eat alive, you feel alive!

Chapter 2

SWEET FRUITS

Note: *The seasons given in the descriptions of the fruits and vegetables apply to the Northern Hemisphere.*

Apple—There are more than 150 varieties of apples in cultivation. Apples are one of the most healthy, simple and pure foods. "An apple a day keeps the doctor away" is a popular saying, meaning that apples contain certain compounds that help maintain health, clean the teeth, and satisfy the appetite.

The apple can be one of your top ten most eaten foods. They can be easily brought along to work or on trips. They are so easy to eat, and do not make a mess like juicier fruits sometimes do. Another reason to eat plenty of apples is that organic apples are available in almost any health food store. Organic apples are even sometimes available in regular markets. Beware of non-organic apples, as they are heavily sprayed and waxed.

There are many varieties of apples in cultivation, so do not just limit yourself to the common "Red Delicious." The best varieties are often the tart ones, or sweet-tart, such as the Baldwin, Fuji, Cortland, Empire, and Gravenstein varieties. Select apples that are firm and vibrantly colored. You can often judge an apple by smell, but sometimes good apples do not have a distinct smell. Make sure they do not feel greasy, as this often means that they have been waxed. Bruises and imperfections do not matter, and may be a good sign! Organic apples do not look as "perfect" as the non-organic ones that often look more like a decoration than they do a real food.

Health benefits: Apples are one of the best fruits, mainly because they contain a moderate amount of sugar that does not rush into the blood stream too quickly. They have plenty of fiber, which acts as a broom in the intestines, insuring good bowel movements. Apples contain malic acid, which cleanses the liver, and helps to maintain healthy bacterial activity in the intestines. They also contain pectin, which helps to prevent the putrefaction of protein.

Season: August (early apples) through May Apples store extremely well.

Season: pricot—Ripe apricots are hard to find in the stores. Unripe apricots can be starchy and give you indigestion. When you are able to find truly ripe apricots, preferably right from the tree, go for it! Ripe apricots are excellent in fruit salads, blended into smoothies, or simply eaten whole.

You might think that a nearly ripe apricot would ripen at room temperature, much like a pear or avocado, but that is not the case and they need to be purchased fully ripe. A fully ripe apricot is deep golden-orange in color with no trace of green, and slightly soft to the touch. A red tint is also a good sign.

Apricots originate from China, where they are widely cultivated. They are members of the drupe family, along with other stone fruits such as peaches, plums, cherries and almonds (which are a nut).

Health benefits: Apricots are a mild laxative, are rich in beta-carotene, and an excellent source of copper, cobalt, and iron. They are a mineral-rich food that is very useful in cases of blood-related diseases.

Season: Apricots are available from May through August (at best).

Banana—Bananas are one of the few fruits found in stores everywhere in the world. Although they are more likely to be grown in tropical countries, banana trees can be grown anywhere that does not experience freezing temperatures, although it will take much longer before they produce fruit. Bananas are also greenhouse-grown in countries like Iceland.

Bananas are a good food for those transitioning into a raw-vegan diet because bananas are high in sugar (with some starch), and are both filling and satisfying.

We have tried not to include too many bananas in the recipes of this book, because typical bananas are hybridized (do not have seeds), and contain a lot of starchy sugar. But due to the expansion of the organic food movement, many brands of exotic organic bananas are becoming a standard item on the shelves of health food stores.

Culinary speaking, there is nothing like the banana to enhance the flavor and add consistency to a smoothie. They are also good when eaten with other dried fruits, and in fruit salads.

Health benefits: Bananas are an excellent source of potassium, as many people know, and of other minerals and nutrients. They are rich in sugar, and are a good food for the very active person.

Season: Bananas are available all year

Blackberry—Blackberries belong to the same family as the raspberry. There are many varieties both in cultivation and growing wild. The wild varieties are especially delicious, and are found in abundance in temperate regions. You will recognize ripe blackberries with their deep black color, softness, and aromatic smell.

Health benefits: Blackberries are a good blood cleanser. They are rich in many minerals.

Season: May through August (may vary according to the location).

Carob—Carob is a pod-shaped fruit, brown in color, and used mainly as a chocolate substitute. It is sweet but not juicy, and can be eaten fresh as well as in a powdered form. Carob originates from the Mediterranean region of Europe. It is mentioned a few times in the Bible.

If you get the chance, try fresh carob. You will have to pick it from a tree, as it is not sold anywhere that I know of. It is a really satisfying food that fills you and takes care of any chocolate craving. The taste of carob is comparable to chocolate, but it does not contain caffeine, and has more minerals and less fat than chocolate. While chocolate is a stimulant, carob is calming.

Health benefits: Fresh carob pods are the perfect remedy for indigestion, diarrhea, and excessive flatulence. They are rich in calcium, and are perfect for building strong bones.

Season: Fresh carob is in season from September through December

Cherimoya—If there is a fruit that is totally under-rated and under-cultivated in the world, it is the cherimoya. They are a member of the *Annona* family, in which we find the sugar apple, soursop, custard apple, and cherimoya, originating from South America. The cherimoya is usually round-shaped, or shaped like a heart. It is light green in color, and sometimes becomes darker as it ripens. Inside the fruit is a white, sweet flesh, which contains many shiny black inedible seeds. The flesh tastes like a mixture of banana, pineapple, and blueberry. Cherimoyas are grown in California, and can be found in some farmers market, health food stores, and exotic fruit stores. They are usually expensive, but are well worth the price.

Cherimoyas can be bought unripe and left to ripen at room temperature on a sunny windowsill—much like an avocado. To eat them, wait until they yield to gentle pressure, then break them apart in your hands. Eat the white flesh, discarding the peel and seeds. You can also use the flesh in smoothies and fruit salads.

Health benefits: Cherimoyas are high in calcium and many trace minerals.

Season: November through April (sometimes up to June).

Cherry—Is there a more beautiful fruit than a deep red cherry growing in pairs? Its aspect has inspired poets and artists throughout the ages. Cherries are a reminder of spring and all the splendors it brings. Cherries have a short season, so make sure you take full advantage of it, and eat as many as you can while they are available. Cherries originate from Eastern Europe and Asia, and are now grown throughout the world.

Select cherries that are bright, deep in color, and firm, with fresh stems. Avoid those that are too soft. Commercial cherries are heavily sprayed, and are often waxed, so make sure you buy organic cherries. Better yet, plant your own cherry trees.

Health benefits: Cherries are a good detoxifying fruit. I recommend that you try going a few days eating cherries only when they are in season. This will give your digestive system a rest, and make you feel great. This type of fruit fast is especially good to help conditions of gout, arthritis, rheumatism, and acidic stomach upset. Cherries have anti-putrid properties that help combat the effects of excess protein foods. They are rich in iron, as many red (blood) fruits are, and help to build healthy blood.

Season: May through July.

Date—Many people think of dates as a dried fruit. Although they can be dried artificially, they are naturally low in water, and do not need to be dried after being picked. However, many date distributors dry them further artificially, and then preserve them in glucose. The best dates are the juiciest ones, the ones available fresh at the stores in season. These soft ripe dates are exquisite compared to the dried dates most people are familiar with.

Good dates should still be moist, and not entirely dried. They should be plump with a shiny skin. Watch out for a fermented aroma, as this is a sign that the dates have spoiled. To prevent fermentation, dates may be frozen. Date trees grow in areas where temperatures are known to dip a little below the freezing point during the night, so keeping your dates refrigerated is normal for them.

The date is the fruit of a variety of palm tree that grows in desert climates. It is grown throughout the world in countries that enjoy a desert-like climate. In America dates are grown in California and Arizona, where many organic farmers are dedicated to growing the best dates in the world. Did you know that if someone were to plant a date palm for you the day you were born, by the time you would have reached your 18th year, the plant would produce enough food to feed you entirely for the rest of your life? Not that eating dates, and nothing else, would be best, but it is an interesting fact.

The date is a fruit that is very high in sugar, in a form that enters the blood stream quickly, and therefore dates do not agree with people suffering with diabetes, hypoglycemia, or candida. People needing to limit their consumption of sugar should limit their intake of dates.

Health benefits: Because of their high sugar content, dates are a good food for active people. They are also good for people who are transitioning away from sugar and chocolate, as they tend to satisfy us in a way these junk foods did in the past. Dates mixed with coconuts and almonds seem to work very well as a replacement for chocolate and candy. Many health food stores sell natural date "cakes," which are a good choice over any other artificial dessert. Powdered date sugar is available in many health food stores, and is an excellent replacement for, and has more nutrients than, cane sugar.

Season:Fall through Winter

Fig—The fig is one of the most amazing fruits on the planet, and one of the fruits highest in calcium and other minerals. They originate from Mediterranean countries, and are grown in California, Greece, Turkey, and other countries that enjoy a warm climate.

Ripe, fresh figs can be found in many markets, health food stores, and exotic produce stores. Ripe figs are soft and slightly wrinkled. There are several varieties of figs, the most popular being the Black Mission (black-blue) and Calimyrna (yellow-white). Although you may sometimes find fresh figs at the store, nothing compares to the experience of eating a fig right off the tree. If you wait until they are at their most ripe and delicious state, as they just start to wrinkle and dry out on the tree, they will taste like grandmother's best jam.

Health benefits: Figs are one of the sweetest fruits, and therefore constitute an amazing source of energy for active people. They contain more mineral matter than most other fruits. They are especially abundant in calcium, which make them a very alkaline fruit. They are excellent as a natural laxative. Their high mucin content and tiny seeds help clean toxins and mucus out of the system. Some studies indicate that figs help to kill pernicious bacteria while promoting the growth of friendly bacteria in the intestines. Dried figs eaten in moderation, (organic and non-sulfured) are also good when fresh figs are not available.

Season: August through November

Grape—The grape is actually a berry growing on vines. Grapes have been grown for thousands of years in Mediterranean countries, and are now grown throughout the world. The varieties that are grown for making wine are usually not the same as those grown for eating. The leaves are edible, and may be marinated in water, soy sauce, or lemon juice, and used to wrap guacamole, nut pâtés, or other raw concoctions.

Grapes are one of the most cleansing fruits, and one abundant in minerals and vitamins. Choose plump fruit still attached to the stem. Color is important, so look for brighter colored fruit. Buy the seeded varieties, and avoid the seedless varieties, which have been developed by humans.

Wine is the result of fermenting raw grape juice. If no preservatives are added, wine can be considered a living food. Research shows that a little wine reduces the levels of cholesterol in the blood, and offers other health benefits. However, new research shows that the benefits might come from certain compounds found in grapes, and that we could get the same benefits from just eating the grapes. Whatever beneficial effects wine may have are overruled by the effects of the alcohol, which is a poison to the system. If you drink wine, make sure that it is organic and free of added sulfites. All wine has naturally occurring sulfites, but some wine-makers add additional sulfites.

Health benefits: Grapes are a very cleansing fruit. High quality seeded grapes rank at the top of the list as a medicinal food. The grape cure used to be very popular in Europe, and consisted of eating only grapes for 1 to 4 weeks. Many people have benefited from this fast. Grape seeds are rich in antioxidants, and can be chewed along with the grapes. Antioxidants, as you may know, are the super-heroes that fight free radicals, the little beasties that wreak havoc on our cells, and play a role in cancer and other degenerative diseases.

Season: July through November.

Grapefruit—While most people are familiar with grapefruits, many have not enjoyed them in their pure state. The way many people eat grapefruits is halved with a spoonful of sugar sprinkled on top. The way raw-vegans eat grapefruit is the way most people eat an orange—by tearing off the rind, and eating the perfectly proportioned sections. The trick to grapefruits is to let them sit for a week or two before eating them either on a sunny windowsill or in a safe place outdoors. They do not go bad quickly, and the extra ripening time allows for the rind to become firmer, and thus easier to tear off.

Health benefits: Grapefruits have powerful cleansing effects, and are especially good to get rid of inorganic calcium deposits in the body (as in arthritis) that result from the over-consumption of grain products and meat. It is a good fruit for those who have a hard time controlling their sugar level.

Season: Winter and early Spring, but they are available all year round.

Kiwi—Kiwis were not well known until the 1970's when they began to be imported from New Zealand. They originate from China, and are now widely grown in California. Named after the Kiwi bird of New Zealand, these fuzzy fruits are commonly used in fruit salads, but are also good eaten by themselves. While it is common to peel the skin off of kiwis, some people eat them whole, skin and all. Ripe kiwis yield to gentle pressure. Organic kiwis have a much better taste than chemically grown kiwis, which are sprayed heavily.

Health benefits: Kiwis contain enzymes that help aid in digestion. They also are one of the richest sources of vitamin C.

Season: November through April.

Lemon—The lemon originated in China or India, and is now grown in warmer climates throughout the world. Used for their juice, lemons are an indispensable ingredient in the raw food cuisine. Use them freshly squeezed on many dishes and salads, or in water. Select lemons that are semi-soft and feel "full" and heavy, with a bright yellow color. Do not be afraid to purchase lemons that are large or oddly shaped these are likely to be of a less hybridized variety.

Health benefits: Lemons are important tools for detoxification, acting like solvent and dissolving mucus in the body. Drink one or two glasses of water with lemon squeezed in it every morning. This will help your body continue its cleansing actions that it was active doing during the night.

Season: Winter and Spring, but they are available all year round.

Lime—Because of their flavor, I prefer limes to lemons. When left to ripen long enough on the trees, limes become yellow. Although they are good green, their flavor is amazing when they are fully ripe (yellow). Limes that fall off the tree usually have a circular "burnt" tint at the bottom. This is a sign that they were allowed to fully ripen on the tree. Select limes that are closer to yellow in color. The use of limes is the same as lemons.

Health benefits: Same as lemons.

Season: Winter and early Spring, but available all year when imported from various locations.

Loquat—The loquat is a little spring fruit growing in California and other sunny climates. We are starting to see it more frequently in the fruit markets.

It originates from Asia where it is more popular. The reason it has not been popular in markets elsewhere is because it is a tender fruit that needs special care during the picking and shipping stages.

Loquats at their prime ripe stage are really delicious. They have a flavor similar to grapes or pineapple. Ripe fruit are yellow-orange; the more bright in color the better. The skin of the fruit also tends to wrinkle while sitting on the tree, as the fruit starts to dry. Fruits in that stage are particularly sweet.

Health benefits: They are supposed to halt vomiting.

Season: May through June.

Mango—The mango is the world's most popular fruit. More children in the world know the word "mango" than "apple." They have been cultivated as far back as eight thousands years ago. The mango tree can reach an enormous size, and bear fruit for decades. Mangos are now starting to become popular in markets in America and Europe. As their popularity grows, their price is becoming more reasonable. Because of the increasing demand for this fruit, it is seen on store shelves throughout the world.

Mangos are a truly magical, sensual, paradisiacal fruit and they come in many sizes, shapes, and colors. The typical mango is about 1/2 to 1 pound, (225-450 grams). Ripe mangos yield to gentle pressure, and emit a very aromatic fragrance. I have found that the best way to select a good mango is by smelling it. Choosing by color is not always best, because there are some varieties that stay green even when they are ripe.

Health benefits: Because mangos are packed with both water and nutrients, they are useful for the kidneys, and as a general blood cleanser. They are a high energy fruit, and perfect for active people and children.

Season: April through September

Melon—Melons belong to the same family as cucumbers and pumpkins, and grow on vines on the ground just like them. If you are one of those who lived all of your life in the city, it is time for you to know that melons do not grow on trees!

There are many types of melon. Among the most popular are the Watermelon, Cantaloupe, Honeydew, Galia, and Persian.

Selecting a perfect melon is not an easy task for a beginner. Some people use a "tapping" technique to determine if a melon is ripe. The idea is to tap the melon, and listen for the sound it makes. If it sounds hollow, or like you are hitting a jug of water, it is ripe. If it does not resonate more; it is not quite ripe. But personally, I think the best way to determine a good melon is by the smell and color. They should have a large white spot that indicates that the fruit has been sitting on the ground for a while. Also, the part where it was connected to the vine should give a little when you press on it.

There are also a lot of people who claim that melons should be eaten alone and not mixed with any other fruit. The idea comes from the food combining theory of Herbert Shelton that has been popularized in the book **Fit for Life**. Believers of this theory should read Dr. Shelton's work more carefully, to find that he actually said: "I have tried eating melons with fresh fruits, and there seems to be no reason why they may not be eaten together, if this is desired."

Health benefits: Melons are the perfect cleanser, and an excellent fruit for detoxification. They are rich in highly mineralized, distilled, organic water, and are ideal for hydrating the body during the hot summer months. They are excellent for people suffering from heart disease, because melons contain some compounds that help thin the blood. Another good thing about melons is that they require hardly any digestion. They pass quickly through the stomach and into the intestines for assimilation. They are no burden on the body, and are great for a mono-diet, during a detoxifying program, and as a food to start eating after a fast.

Season: Summer and early Fall.

Mulberry—The mulberry is the fruit of a shrub or tree that grows in many temperate climates. They have an incredible flavor when fully ripe, and are highly prized by birds, who often get them before humans do. They vary in size and color, as they can be white, black, purple, or red (sometimes two or three colors are seen on one berry). Selecting good mulberries is quite simple: they must be as bright, and as deep in color as possible, and soft.

Health benefits: They are high in iron, calcium, and many other minerals. They are a good food for helping stomach ulcers.

Season: June through August.

Nectarine—Nectarines are a popular fruit during the summer months in America and Europe. They are similar to the peach, but without the fuzzy skin, and with a flavor that some people prefer. There are many varieties, but the best ones are the white nectarines, which have a sweet white flesh. Good, ripe nectarines are slightly soft and give a sweet, fragrant aroma. They may also be purchased semi-hard, and left to ripen at room temperature on a windowsill. Commercial nectarines are rarely good as they are picked too early. For the best taste, look for tree-ripened nectarines. You are more likely to find them at a farmer's market.

Health benefits: Nectarines are rich in beta-carotene, and are an excellent digestive aid.

Season: June through August.

Orange—Oranges are native to China. They come in many varieties that are available throughout the year, mainly during the winter. The best oranges, sweet and delicious, are those that are kept longest on the tree to ripen. They might not look as "perfect" as other oranges, as they may be bruised and wrinkled, but they definitely have the fullest flavor.

The most common varieties of oranges include: **Navel**, the most popular that is available in the winter, and good to eat by simply tearing off the rind and eating the perfectly proportioned pieces one by one. **Valencia**, the variety that comes into season in the Fall, is used mainly for juicing, although they are also excellent to eat by hand. **Blood Oranges** are another really good variety of orange. You will recognize them by their skin spotted with tints of red and purple. The flesh of the blood orange is also tinted red or purple, and they have a tangy raspberry aftertaste. They are quite popular in Mediterranean countries. The *season* for blood oranges is *December through June.*

Health benefits: Oranges are high in calcium, and are a good body cleanser. The acids they contain help dissolve mucus in the body. Many people have used oranges on a mono-diet, either in juice or by itself, as a way to detoxify.

When going on such a program, remember that you should not eat too many oranges, as an excess of their acids may create problems. If you are doing the orange juice fast, dilute the juice with pure distilled water.

Season: Fall, Winter and Spring.

Papaya—The high life-force of papayas can be observed by the incredible speed that the seeds sprout and grow into a tree. It is common for papaya trees that are less than a year old to bear fruit. Papayas taste like a cantaloupe, but can have a consistency close to custard, and a very unique, musky flavor. They have been called the melons of the tropics.

Papayas originate from Central America, and are now grown all around the world in tropical climates. At the store, you will find basically two varieties: the smaller, yellowish Hawaiian papaya, and the bigger, orange-colored, Mexican papaya. Some people think that the small Hawaiian papaya has a better flavor than the Mexican one. This is not always true, as you can find really good Mexican papayas when they are truly ripe. Select a good papaya judging by its color. The deeper the color—yellow or orange—the better Mexican papayas turning almost red-orange are really good. They are soft when ripe, and yield to gentle pressure. You can buy the fruit when it is still firm, and let it ripen at room temperature. Papayas can be found in many fruit markets around the world.

Health benefits: Papayas are a good body cleanser, help reduce gas, eliminate gastric indigestion, soothe irritation and inflammation, and help to cleanse and detoxify the system. They are especially rich in beta-carotene, calcium, and vitamin C. Green papayas are rich in enzymes that aid in breaking down protein. In many countries green papayas are cooked along with meat to tenderize it. You can add small chunks of green papayas (without the skin) to smoothies for an enzyme boost.

Season: All year round.

Passion Fruit—Passion fruits come in several varieties, including purple, sweet, giant, and banana. They grow on a vine, and are native to the Amazon. Passion fruits are about the size and shape of a large egg, and have a tough, cardboard-like shell. As they ripen, the shell becomes more and more wrinkled. As a general rule, the more wrinkled, the better and sweeter it is going to be.

Inside the shell, there is a juicy, slimy, yellow-orange pulp filled with edible seeds about the size of grape seeds. You can poke a hole into the passion fruit and suck the edible part out, seeds and all. Because the seeds are difficult to chew, most people simply swallow them whole. You can also cut it in half and eat it with a spoon. Adding some orange juice makes it particularly delicious. The unique flavor is appealing, musky, guava-like, and sweetish-tart. It is strong, tangy, and really good when at its prime ripe stage.

Health benefits: Passion fruits are an excellent source of iron.

Season: Fall.

Peach—Peaches are native to China, and are now cultivated throughout the world. They are a delicious fruit when ripened on the tree, but unfortunately, they are not often sold in this perfect condition. In some places you may find tree-ripened peaches or, even better, get them directly from the farmer.

Select peaches that are firm and yield to gentle pressure. They should have a really pleasant aroma, and be vibrantly colored. Of course it all depends on the variety, since there are hundreds of them. Personally, I prefer white peaches to any other varieties that I have tried so far.

Health benefits: Peaches are a good diuretic. They are excellent for the complexion and the hair. A natural laxative, they aid in cleansing the system, especially when dealing with kidney and bladder troubles.

Season: June through August.

Pear—Pear or apple? My favorite is apples, but sometimes a perfect pear is hard to beat. Some of the many varieties of pear include: Anjou, a popular winter pear; Bartlett, a summer variety; Bosc, a long, dark yellow, or brownish variety that is super sweet when left to completely ripen (they do not need to be crunchy like everybody thinks); Comice, one of the sweetest and more flavorsome varieties. Chinese or Asian pear is a different type of fruit that has the flavor of a pear (and somewhat of the orange), and the crunchiness of an apple.

Pears will ripen off the tree. If your store does not sell ripe pears, simply purchase unripe ones and let them ripen at room temperature. They are at their peak when they have a creamy texture that dissolves in your mouth.

Health benefits: Pears are good cleansers and valuable for people with sluggish bowels. They are rich in alkaline minerals, and help overcome acidic conditions.

Season: August through April.

Persimmon—Persimmons originate from China, and are starting to be more popular in America. They look like orange tomatoes, and are ready to eat when they are as soft as an overripe tomato. Otherwise they are astringent, and will dry out your mouth faster than anything. In their ripe stage (super soft), they are very sweet, much like jam. The most common variety is called Hachiya.

I must reiterate that persimmons must be eaten super-soft! Softer than you might think. There is one variety, called the Fuyu that can be eaten when crunchy. This variety, however, can still benefit from longer ripening.

You can buy persimmons unripe, and let them ripen at room temperature. To hasten the process, you can place them in a paper bag in a dark, warm spot.

The wild persimmons that grow in some parts of the United States are smaller than the oriental varieties. They are not as juicy, but are sweeter. They have a richness in their sweetness that reminds me of dates.

Health benefits: Persimmons are one of the richest sources of beta-carotene, and tend to have mild laxative properties.

Season: December through February.

Pineapple—Pineapples originate from South America, and are now grown throughout the tropical areas of the world. You probably know how to recognize a pineapple, but do you know what a ripe pineapple looks like? The green pineapples you find in the store certainly do not deserve their name. A ripe pineapple is golden-yellow.

When you purchase a pineapple, look for those imported by aircraft ('jet-imported"), and that are yellow-gold in color. Smell them at the base—they should have a very sweet, aromatic fragrance.

You can eat pineapples plain, add them to salads, or juice them. Maybe you think that pineapples are too acidic. If so, try eating a ripe (yellow) pineapple, and you will realize you can eat much more before feeling that burning sensation in the mouth, which is the pineapple's way of telling you that you have eaten enough. If you eat too much pineapple, you can experience a sore top of your mouth, so be careful, and eat them in moderation.

Health benefits: Pineapples are rich in "bromelin," a protein-digesting enzyme. This is the powerful enzyme that causes the burning in your mouth if you eat too much pineapple. Pineapples are good for digestion, and as a diuretic. They are also very rich in vitamin C.

Season: Available all year round.

Plum and Prune—Plums are another summer fruit that can only be fully appreciated when they have been allowed to ripen on the tree. Most stores sell plums that have been picked prematurely. Plums come in all colors, including red, maroon, black, pink, green and yellow. All of the varieties differ in taste and shape. Select tree-ripened plums that are plump, fully colored and fragrant. The European plum is believed to be native to Asia.

Health benefits: Plums are a laxative and a stimulant. They are a high-energy fruit that is good for the nerves. Because they are rich in some acids (including oxalic acid), it is better to eat plums in moderation. Dried plums are called "prunes." Plums and prunes are a rich source of iron.

Season: June through September

Pomegranate—Pomegranates are native to Persia. They are mentioned in classical mythology, the Bible, and the teachings of Mohammed. They are also featured in the archaeology of Solomon's temple, and in Tarot cards. They are often given as gifts to newly married couples because pomegranates are thought to be good for sexual toning and to promote fertility.

Pomegranates are grown in California, and in many parts of the world with sunny climates. They are a wonderful reddish-brown fruit that is often found dried in art and craft stores where they are sold for use in holiday ornamentation and seasonal decorations. Many people are so used to seeing pomegranates as a decoration that they do not recognize them as a food. While there are miniature pomegranates, the ones that are usually sold for eating are about the size of a large orange. A good quality pomegranate will have a thin, tough, and unbroken skin—a broken skin is indicative of a tree that did not receive enough water, but the fruit may still be good. The inside of a pomegranate contains hundreds of jewel-like, pea-sized, crimson, transparent seeds filled with juice, and that burst at the lightest bite. The juice has a tart flavor that is somewhere between the taste of a cranberry and strawberry. The seeds are good eaten by themselves, or tossed into salads. They also add a wonderful flavor to guacamole. The juice of the seeds may be used in all sorts of dishes, such as puddings, syrups, and marinated vegetables.

To open a pomegranate, cut the crown off, and soak the whole fruit under water for about 15 to 30 minutes. Break the pomegranate open under water and the seeds will fall to the bottom as the pulp floats to the top. To juice the seeds, simply mix them in a blender, then strain the juice to remove the seed casings. Whole pomegranates, or just their seeds, may be refrigerated or frozen. The juice lasts for five days under refrigeration, or six months when frozen, and can be used to make tasty ice cubes.

Health benefits: Pomegranates have been used to treat sore throats, skin inflammations, rheumatism, and dysentery. Scientists in Japan have found pomegranates to be beneficial for women who experience severe menopausal symptoms. Pomegranates have no fat, lots of fiber, and are a good source for a variety of nutrients, including vitamin C and potassium. They have many beneficial trace elements. They contain more antioxidants than grapes, and may be more effective than red wine in preventing heart-related diseases.

Season: July through November

Prickly Pear—Also know as the Panini, or the Cactus fruit, this fruit owns its name for good reasons. It grows on a cactus, and is native to Central America.

It is smaller than a pear, and wears small thorns on its peel. The ones you buy in the markets usually have had their thorns removed, so they can be handled safely. But be cautious nonetheless.

To eat a prickly pear safely, you have to peel them with a knife. You can peel it, or cut it in half, and eat it with a spoon. It tastes similar to a melon, but with many hard seeds inside. Not everyone agrees on what should be done with all these seeds. Some say we should spit them out, others say we can swallow them. I personally choose to swallow them. I guess you should avoid eating too many, so you do not get a blocked intestine.

Prickly Pears usually come in two colors: green or red. They are both good. To choose ripe fruits, look for those that are tender but not squishy. They are best when they have a deep, even color.

Health benefits: Prickly pears are rich in calcium, and are a beneficial food for people with sugar sensitivity problems, because of their low sugar content.

Season: Fall.

Raspberry—Raspberries are a popular berry that are cultivated, but also grow wild in many parts of the world. Most people think all raspberries are red, but there are also black, yellow, and white varieties that may be more delicious than the red variety.

Although you may find quality raspberries in the store, try to get the wild ones if they grow where you live. They are likely to be a lot sweeter and so much better nutritionally than the cultivated varieties. On average, the wild raspberries have more minerals and other nutrients than those grown on farms.

Health benefits: Raspberries are rich in calcium, iron, and other minerals. They are good system cleansers. They can help clear out accumulated mucus in your body, especially when you dedicate a few days to a raspberry cure—eating only berries and drinking water. This should prove to be an interesting experience, as you will save money that would have been spent on store-bought foods, while allowing your system to both rest from food, and work to dispose of accumulated toxins.

Season: July through August.

Strawberry—Strawberries are the most popular of all berries. They are also the most hybridized and rank high on the list of produce grown with pesticides and fertilizers. The wild strawberry is a lot smaller than the cultivated variety, but is often sweeter and, as with all fruits, has much better nutrition than the cultivated one. When purchasing strawberries, judge them by their color and smell. They should be deep red, and have a wonderful aroma. Avoid the ones with green or white tips, as well as the overly large, super hybridized varieties. And, of course, always purchase organically grown strawberries.

Health benefits: Strawberries are renowned as a skin-cleansing food. They are a rich source of vitamin C.

Season: Summer

Tangerine—Tangerines are a delicious citrus fruit, usually much tastier than oranges. Tangerines peel easily, and have a wonderful flavor that is more rounded, but similar to the taste of oranges. Good tangerines have lots of seeds in them, which is always a sign of a good, healthy citrus fruit.

If you like their flavor better, feel free to use tangerines for the recipes in this book where oranges are listed as an ingredient.

Health benefits: Same as oranges.

Season: Winter.

Watermelon—Although watermelons are no different than other melons, I thought they should be discussed separately as they are truly the queen of all melons. Watermelons are without a doubt the ultimate refreshment during the hot summer months.

They are native to the tropical regions of Africa.

During the past few years, many watermelons sold in stores are of a human-altered seedless variety. This hybridized version is nothing to be proud of. Seedless fruits tend to be unbalanced in minerals and high in sugar. Seedless fruits do not taste as good, and have no nutritional advantage over seeded fruits especially with the watermelon, as its seeds are actually nutritious.

Health benefits: Watermelons are cooling and hydrating. Their high-quality water is useful in cleansing the digestive and blood systems. They are a powerful diuretic, which will help wash the bladder out in no time. Watermelon juice is often indicated in many detoxification programs. The rind can be juiced with the fruit to lower the sugar content of the juice.

Season: Summer

Chapter 3
OTHER TROPICAL FRUITS

There are many tropical and exotic fruits worth trying. The following fruits are very popular in some countries, but are not well known in the Western world. I have been able to find all of them in Asian markets, and in specialty stores in the United States and Canada. To find these fruits, ask the people who work in the produce section, especially in stores where you have seen fruits that you are not familiar with. Ask which fruit they are, and what they taste like. Also ask about any other unusual fruits that you may see available. The people in the produce section are frequently excellent sources of information about how to eat the various fruits that they sell.

Carambola—This fruit originates from Sri Lanka and the Moluccas, and has been cultivated in Asia for a long time. It now grows in many tropical countries. The fruit is 3 to 6 inches long (7 to 15 centimeters), and its waxy skin turns yellow-orange when ripe. Inside there are only a few seeds and the fruit is eaten with its skin. It is very juicy, sweet, and slightly acidic. It is also called "starfruit" because when the fruit is cut into slices, the slices thus obtained look like stars, and these are wonderful for decorating fruit salads and desserts.

Dragon Fruit—The Spanish name for the Dragon Fruit is pitahaya, and it originates from Nicaragua. You can often find these fruits in Asian markets. Dragon Fruit is definitely one of the most beautiful fruits. Depending on the variety, it may be red or yellow, and as large as a big mango. The fruit must still be firm when ripe. If you wait until it is soft, it will no longer be good. To prepare, you simply cut it in half, and eat the inside flesh with a spoon. The edible part is white, juicy, and has a very delicate taste. There are many small seeds about the size of those found in a kiwi, which are also eaten. The center of the fruit is the sweetest part.

Eggfruit—The proper name for this fruit is "canistel," but it is more often called "eggfruit." Some also call it "yellow sapote," or "canistel sapote." It is native to southern Mexico and Central America. The fruit is usually oval, and the size of a small apple. When ripe, the skin turns yellow-orange, and the fruit becomes very soft. It can be eaten with the skin, but is most commonly eaten peeled. The edible part of the fruit is creamy, very sweet, and has a texture similar to that of a boiled egg, which is how it got its name. Because of its high sugar content, it is one of the most high-caloric fruits.

Feijoa—The feijoa tree is native to South America, and is now grown commercially in California and New Zealand. It is also called the "pineapple guava," because the inside of the fruit tastes like a juicy, pineapple-flavored guava. It can be shaped like an egg or more elongated, and is green in color like an olive. Ripe fruits are soft and their skin is not edible. If they are not ripe, you can let them ripen at room temperature. You will know when the fruit is ripe because it has an enticing aroma. To eat it, you can break it apart with your hands, or cut it in length, and eat the delicious flesh inside.

Guava—The guava could be called the apple of the tropics. There it grows wild in abundance because birds everywhere drop the seeds. It is native to South America, but is now grown throughout the world. There are many varieties of guavas, but the most common variety is round, strongly perfumed, and cream- like in color (but which can also be pink, red, yellow, or other bright colors when ripe). The flesh holds an abundance of seeds that are swallowed. The skin is very thin and is usually eaten with the fruit. Ripe guavas are soft and perfumed, unripe ones are green and hard. Small guavas also exist that are the size of a small plum. The strawberry guava is one of the smaller varieties.

Lichis—There are many ways to spell the name of this fruit: litchi, lychee, lichee, laiche, etc. But any way it is spelled; it refers to the same fruit. The lichi fruit is smaller than a walnut, with a hard, scaly, bright-red outer covering that hides its translucent white flesh surrounding a dark, shiny seed. The edible part tastes like a grape. Its fragrance makes me think that it tastes like how a rose smells. The usual way people eat lichis is out of a can at a Chinese restaurant. If you have tried them that way, and did not like them, do not give up because lichis are truly one of the most delicious fruits in existence. In China they are considered the most luscious of all fruits. They have been grown for thousands of years in Asia, where many meals are accompanied with lichis. You may find fresh lichis during the summer at Asian markets, or other fruit markets. Good ripe lichis should be plump, with a tight skin, and not cracked. They go bad quickly, and you will often find some fermented ones amongst a bunch of good ones. The smell should be your best guide.

Longan—The longan tree belongs to the same family as the lichi and rambutan. It is believed to have originated in India, and is now widely cultivated in Asia, where it is extremely popular. Longans are about the same size as lichis, but their skin is free of studs. Inside there is a white, translucent flesh surrounding a dark seed. It has a taste similar to lichis, but with a muskier undertone. Longans are usually sold attached to the branch. To select good fresh ones, make sure they are not too soft. They are best eaten on their own, or added to fruit salads.

Mamey—This fruit is native to South America, where it is very popular in some countries. There are many varieties. It can be the size of an orange or larger, and the flesh inside is melting and juicy. The taste is similar to pumpkin pie. You open it like a mango, and can use the edible part in fruit salads, or to eat on its own. It is rich in many vitamins and minerals, including iron.

Mangosteen—This fruit originates from Indonesia, and has been cultivated for thousands of years. It is about the size of a tangerine. It has a thick, dark skin, which protects the translucent white segments inside. The taste and texture of this edible part is very delicate. It melts in the mouth, with an acid-sweet flavor that is divine. To open the fruit, use a knife to cut a circle around the middle, and open the top part, leaving the segments exposed in their natural container.

Rambutan—Native to the southeast Asian jungles, this fruit is closely related to the lichi. It is about the same size, but with a reddish tint, and is covered with long "hairs." Inside there is a translucent, juicy, white aromatic flesh similar to the lichi, but more acidic. It is best eaten on its own, or mixed in fruit salads.

Sapodilla—This fruit originates from Mexico and Central America. It looks like a small mango, but its skin is brownish. The fruit must yield to a gentle touch, much like an avocado, before being opened and eaten. Inside there is a brownish, juicy, melting flesh that is very sweet, and that has a flavor that reminds one of maple syrup. A few inedible, shiny, dark seeds are found in the middle. Sapodilla is best mixed in fruit salads, as its strongly sweet flavor may not appeal to everybody. But its high sugar content is appropriate for very active persons.

Sapote—Native to Central America, sapotes (pronounce Sa-Po-Tay's) are now grown throughout Latin America, Hawaii, and California, as well as in many countries that enjoy a hot climate. Sapotes come in many varieties. First there is white sapote which, when fully ripe, tastes like vanilla custard. There is also a black sapote, which tastes like chocolate pudding. All varieties of this fruit are about the size of an apple or smaller. They have a thin skin, which protects the juicy, sweet, melting flesh, and emit a wonderful aroma when fully ripe. Because of its fragility, it is impossible to ship the fruit in the ripe stage. It almost breaks apart in your hands when fully ripe. Most sapotes sold are picked green, and, because of this, do not have the amazing flavor a tree-ripened sapote possesses. But if you have the chance to live or travel where sapotes grow, do not miss trying this wonderful fruit.

Soursop—This is another fruit that is native to South America, and one that is now widely cultivated in Asia, as well as many tropical countries throughout the world. The size of the fruit ranges from as small as a mango to as large as a football. It may weigh as much as 10 pounds. The skin is green, and has a leathery appearance. The fruit must yield to gentle pressure to be ripe. Inside you will find an amazing number of small black seeds bathing in a sweet-acid white flesh that tastes similar to a pineapple. The way I like to eat soursop is to cut the bottom and top of the fruit with a knife so that you can easily peel the skin off, leaving only a big, white, fleshy fruit. Then remove the seeds one by one, and put the white flesh in a separate bowl. This is a lengthy process, but worth the time spent. Then, once you have separated all of the white flesh from the seeds, you put all of the flesh into a blender and liquefy it. This creates a delicious cream that can be eaten with a spoon. In Asia they add milk to this preparation.

Sugar Apple—This is the English name given to a fruit that is native to South America. It can also be called "sweetsop," as opposed to the fruit called "soursop." The sugar apple belongs to the same family as the cherimoya, but has a different appearance. It is round, ovoid, about the size of an apple, and its skin is composed of knobby segments, often with a reddish tint. The inside looks similar to the cherimoya, with a sweet white flesh in which bathe many black seeds, but it is sweeter than the cherimoya, and has a slightly different flavor that is similar to rose water. It is usually eaten on its own, or mixed in fruit salads. It is rich in vitamins and minerals, including calcium.

Chapter 4

NON-SWEET FRUITS

WHAT IS A FRUIT?

Many of us think that fruits are the juicy, sweet gifts from the trees described in the previous chapter. But, as you will discover, the realm of fruit is much more vast than bananas and oranges. Did you know, for example, that pumpkins are a fruit? Did you know that avocados are also a fruit? Olives too? Yes, all of these and many more are fruits.

A fruit is a food that carries within itself the seeds for the reproduction of the plant. Fruits come from a flower, and by strict definition, fruit is the ripened ovary of a female flower. We like to think of fruit as a symbiotic relation between the plant and the fruit eaters. The tree (or the plant) wants to spread its seeds far and wide. So, instead of just producing seeds, it decides to wrap these seeds in some tasty and nutritious package. Then the fruit eaters come along, get attracted to the fruits, carry them around to eat them, and thus spread the seeds far and wide. If the seeds are swallowed, as in the case with the small edible seeds of tomatoes, figs, and other fruits, they are then carried even farther as they are transported in the intestines of the fruit-eating animal, and later released intact through the feces.

Most humans today do not have the same relation with fruit trees as their ancestors. Fruits are now predominantly grown on farms, picked by under-paid workers, sold at stores, bought by consumers and, after eaten, the seeds of the fruits are usually thrown into the garbage.

Some of the happiest people I have met are farmers who grow fruit trees using natural methods. I see them radiating an aura of peace and oneness with the Earth. I think this is because their life and sustenance revolves around what their trees produce—which is in direct relation to the blessings of Nature. I believe that it is good to go back to the days when we were more in tune with Nature and the goodness of the Earth. One way to do so is to grow our own gardens where we, like the fruit farmers, can learn how dependent we are on Nature. Planting, caring for, and enjoying the bounties of a garden, big or small, is something everyone should experience.

Cucumber—Although most people think of cucumbers as a vegetable (probably because they are used to eating them in salads), the cucumber is actually the fruit of a vine (like melons and squash). Cucumbers are especially refreshing in the summer, as their high water and low sugar content is perfect for hot weather. They are native to India and Egypt. There are basically three varieties of cucumbers: the long thin variety used in salads; the shorter, thicker, slicing cucumber also used in salads; and the small round one, used for pickling, but that is also excellent eaten raw.

Select a good cucumber by looking for firm, brightly-colored ones. Try out different varieties, and strive to find organically grown cucumbers. Cucumbers are one of the most heavily sprayed fruits and frequently waxed.

Health benefits: Cucumbers are a cooling alkaline fruit that also possess diuretic properties. Eating lots of cucumbers is known to facilitate excretion of wastes through the kidneys, and helps to dissolve uric acid accumulations, such as kidney and bladder stones. Their high potassium content makes them useful in dealing with conditions of high and low blood pressure.

Season: Summer and early Fall.

Eggplant—Like the tomato and pepper, the eggplant is a member of the nightshade family. It is called "aubergine" in France and the United Kingdom. The fruit is usually only eaten cooked. I have one use for it raw: you can marinate it in nama shoyu or tamari sauce, and create a raw "lasagna" **(See the book "Easy Gourmet Raw Food Cuisine)**. Eggplants are believed to be native to South Central Asia, and possibly India. There exist many varieties, ranging from as small as an egg to as large as a football. The most common varieties in the United States are large and purple.

Health benefits: Eggplants are rich in bioflavanoids, which help renew arteries and prevent cardiovascular diseases. Eggplants are mostly water, and therefore, very cleansing.

Season: Summer and early Fall

Okra—Okra is a fruit that originates from North Africa. ft was introduced into the United States about one hundred years ago. It is very common in the south of the United States, as it is eaten cooked in some southern concoctions. When raw, it is slimy in consistency.

Health benefits: Raw okra is rich in silicon, which is useful for the skin and bones.

Season: Summer and Fall.

Pepper—Peppers are native to South America. There are basically two types of peppers: bell peppers (sweet, mild peppers), and hot peppers (chile peppers). Both types of pepper come in different colors, but keep in mind that most green peppers are unripe. As the peppers ripen on the plant they become red, yellow or orange. But some peppers remain green even when ripe. The red (yellow or orange) peppers usually have a higher vitamin C content than green peppers.

Sweet bell peppers can be used in salads and other dishes, or eaten on their own, while hot chile peppers are used to spice a variety of dishes. Chile peppers come in many varieties, the most popular being jalapeño. Cayenne peppers are dried and dehydrated into a powder that is used as a spice. Whenever I use hot peppers in my recipes, I refer to jalapeno or cayenne powder. Feel free to use any type of pepper that you desire, to the degree of heat that you enjoy. Also, be careful when handling hot peppers. Remember to always wash your hands thoroughly afterwards.

Health benefits: Both sweet and hot peppers are rich in Vitamin C (up to six times as much as oranges). They also contain Vitamin B, which aids in food absorption, and normalizes the brain and nervous system. Hot peppers are antibacterial and stimulants. The active substance in peppers that gives them their bite is capsaicin, which stimulates the body to heal and cleanse. It helps clear parasites out of the intestines, normalizes blood pressure, improves the circulatory system, increases peristaltic movement, and helps the capillaries, arteries, and veins to gain more elasticity. Chile peppers are a wonderful medicine to take during the first months of your change in diet. You can juice them along with your vegetable juices, or add them to salads, salsas, and guacamole.

Season: Summer through Fall.

Tomato—The tomato is the most famous member of the nightshade family. It is native to South America, and is now eaten throughout the world. The fruit has been hybridized terribly, to the point where many tomatoes now found in stores are incredibly tasteless. Organic and homegrown tomatoes are always tastier than those sold in stores. There are many good varieties, most of which can only be found in home gardens. This is a good reason to consider growing your own tomatoes. They are quite easy to grow—you just need a sunny spot. When the season is over, and you have green tomatoes still hanging on the plant, you can pick them, wrap them individually in newspaper, and put them into a box. They will ripen, taking from a few weeks to a few months. When selecting tomatoes at the store, choose firm, plump ones, with a vibrant color. Avoid commercial tomatoes, as they are most likely to be genetically engineered, and chemically grown.

Health benefits: Tomatoes are a great mineralized, high water content food. But as with all members of the nightshade family, it is wise to not eat too many tomatoes, or at least to not eat them everyday, because of their oxalic acid content. Oxalic acid is an acid found in some fruits and vegetables which hinders the absorption of calcium. It is nothing to be feared—as it is only the abuse of the foods rich in this acid that creates a problem. However, people suffering from arthritic conditions should avoid foods from the nightshade family completely. This includes eggplant, potatoes, tomatoes, and peppers.

Season: Summer and early Fall.

Squash—Squash is an abundant fruit that grows on a vine, and comes in an incredible array of varieties—as many varieties as there are shapes. Squash is traditionally eaten steamed, baked, or cooked in stir-fries, mixed into casseroles, and used in soups. You will probably only want to eat the tastiest varieties in the living, raw state. Some popular varieties include banana squash, yellow squash, spaghetti squash, butternut squash, and zucchini. Zucchini may be the most popular member of the squash family, and is the most common type of squash used in the raw food cuisine. We use zucchini to make raw "pasta," as explained in my book **Easy Gourmet Raw Food Cuisine.** Zucchinis are called "courgettes" in England, which is actually the French word for this fruit, meaning "little squash."

Health Benefits: Squash, as a highly alkaline, high water content food, are an excellent remedy for acidosis of the liver and the blood. Seeds of squash are helpful in expelling roundworms and tapeworms.

Season: Summer Fall, Winter

Chapter 5
FATTY FRUITS

Avocado—A staple in the raw food diet. Although many people consider them to be a member of the vegetable family, they are truly a fruit. The avocado trees originate from Guatemala, where they can still be found growing wild.

Many varieties of avocados are in cultivation. Do not limit yourself to Hass. If you can find other varieties, such as Fuerte, Reed, or Pinkerton, try them. Even if avocados can be purchased unripe and left to ripen at room temperature, you must understand that they are often picked too early, without letting the full oil content set in. Mature avocados are more bruised and imperfect-looking than immature ones. Sometimes immature avocados may be identified with a reddish tint on them, or a tendency to wrinkle without ripening. A good, mature avocado becomes quite fatty and can be enjoyed without seasonings. Ripe avocados yield to gentle pressure.

Health benefits: The avocado is a rich source of essential fatty acids. They are also rich in vitamin E.

Season: Depends on the variety. With different varieties overlapping each other they can be found all year round.

Durian—This is a fruit you probably have never heard of, and will probably be quite amazed when you see it for the first time. Imagine a roundish-shaped fruit, the size of a soccer ball, brown-gold in color, and covered with little spikes. Some people think it smells like rotten cheese, but tastes like vanilla custard. Although the smell of durian is quite strong and unusual, I do not consider it to be bad. In fact I like it.

Many people agree that eating a durian is one of the most intense food experiences you can have, although most cannot quite figure out how to eat it. First you should know where to get it.

Durian is grown in Thailand and Malaysia, where it is prized. In the Western world, it is imported and is commonly available in Asian markets in most cities.

There are basically three types of durian products available in stores. Fresh, whole-frozen, and package-frozen. Fresh durian is only available a few months a year (usually in the summer), and quite expensive. Expect to pay $20-$40 for one whole fruit. But it is worth it. Frozen durian is available all year round. It is picked ripe, and frozen whole. You will have to thaw it for 8-24 hours before eating. You may also find packaged durian, which is fresh, frozen durian flesh with no seeds, in a plastic container.

You might not like durian the first time you try it. This may be because you need to acquire a taste for it, or simply because you got a bad one. Selecting a good durian is not an easy task. So you may want to ask the people at the Asian market to pick a good one for you. If you want to try to pick one yourself, aim for those that are smaller and somewhat heavy for their size. The color should be more yellowish than greenish and the thorns large—the larger the thorns, the smaller the seeds. Try to squeeze two thorns together—it should be easy to do. There should also be a faint aroma of bittersweet butterscotch and almond with a bouquet of wild honey. Overripe durians split along lines of natural weakness which are faintly visible among the spines. To open a durian, insert a stout knife into such a line. Durians have about five segments, each containing several large seeds and the creamy custard-like flesh.

Health benefits: The durian is rich in essential fatty acids, high quality protein, and is reputed to be an aphrodisiac.

Season: All seasons, depending on the location.

Olive—Olives are a biblical fruit associated in the scriptures with symbols of goodness, happiness, purity and prosperity. In ancient Greece during the height of their culture Solon, the great lawgiver, enacted laws protecting all olive trees. He made it a capital offense to kill a tree or cut one down. The Romans were the first to perfect the stone-press with which they extracted the olive's oil. The Romans believed the olive to be an incredibly sexual fruit, an aphrodisiac—especially when eaten in large quantities.

Olives are usually picked green (unripe), and then pickled in a solution of water and salt (as a preservative). They can also be picked black (ripe), and left to dry in the sun. Most olives you find in stores have vinegar added, but it is possible to find some without it. Sun-dried olives have salt on them.

Olive trees are ubiquitous in the southwestern United States (California, Arizona and Nevada) as well as throughout the Mediterranean world, the Middle East, and India.

Health benefits: The olive is high in minerals, especially calcium. It is also rich in vitamin A and E. Olive oil can be used externally.

Season: Olives are available all year round, but are picked in the Fall, because this is when they are ripe.

Chapter 6
DRIED FRUITS

Fruits can be dried under the sun or in a dehydrator, and then stored for long periods of time in a cool, dry place. Although the dehydration process damages or destroys some nutrients, fruits and vegetables that have been dried at a low heat still retain some raw vitality. Thus dried fruits can be used during the long months of winter, when most fresh fruits are not available. Dried fruits constitute a source of concentrated energy, and should be eaten in moderation due to their high sugar content. Dried fruits may be used to create a variety of delicious living desserts that I include in Chapter 20.

When buying dried fruits, make sure they are organic and non-sulfured. Sulfur is an unhealthy chemical that is used in the preservation of commercial dried fruit for monetary reasons, as sulfured fruits are juicier and look better (according to the industry's standards). For example, the sulfured apricots you will find in the stores are those bright orange ones. Experiments conducted by Dr. H.W. Wiley, former chief chemist of the United States Department of Agriculture, demonstrated that the use of sulfurous acid in food is always harmful. It degenerates the kidneys, retards the formation of red corpuscles, and destroys the vitamins in the fruit. Real organic dried apricots are more brownish in color. The label should mention: non-sulfured. All dried fruits may be bought through the mail, from one of the companies listed in Appendix 4.

COMMONLY USED DRIED FRUITS

Apricot—Some of the best sun-dried organic apricots come from Turkey. They are moist and sweet, and form a good little snack during the winter. Other excellent varieties are grown all over the world, including in California.

Raisin—The most popular dried fruit, raisins are now made using seedless grapes. Raisins used to have seeds inside of them, which added to their flavor and nutrition. But since humans have altered the plants, people have gotten used to eating raisins that lack seeds. About the only way you will get the best quality raisins is to dehydrate seeded grapes yourself.

Fig—Figs are a popular dried fruit. They are not too sweet, and have little seeds that give figs an interesting crunchy consistency when eaten. They grow all over the warmer climates, so there is always a fresh supply. They should be stored in a cool, dry place so that they do not ferment, or accumulate mold. They are rich in calcium, and are helpful for freeing constipation.

Prune—Some varieties of plums are cultivated to be dried as prunes. I believe they are the best of all dried fruits. Prunes are preferable to dates or other dried fruits because of their mineral content, and the fact that you will be less prone to overeat them, without facing some consequences. Although it is true that prunes act as a laxative for some people, I have found that when you have been on a raw food diet for long enough, you can eat a reasonable amount of them with no worries.

Other Dried Fruits Include: apples, blueberries, cherries, mangos, mulberries, olives, papayas, pineapples, and tomatoes.

Chapter 7

VEGETABLES

Artichoke—Artichokes are eaten cooked, and rarely raw. If they are very young, they can be eaten raw with delight. There is only a small edible part at the base of each leaf, as well as the base of the vegetable. You will have to cut it in half with a knife, in order to reach the good part. Artichokes are native to the Mediterranean.

Jerusalem Artichoke (also called sunchoke) is a different plant than the artichoke above. It is a plant native to North America that is eaten for its knobby root. It is similar to the potato, but much less starchy. They can be eaten sliced, or grated in salads and coleslaw, with a raw mayonnaise.

Health Benefits: Artichokes are diuretic, while sunchokes are good for diabetic people.

Season: Fall and Winter

Asparagus—Asparagus is native to Europe, and now grows wild in North America and many other places. The spears can be eaten raw. Select them when they are young, fresh, sweet and tender. They should be bright green, straight, firm, and not too thick. The part that is good to eat is the tip, as the base is often too fibrous. You will find that they are a diuretic, and leave a distinct smell in the urine.

Health benefits: Because of a substance called "asparagine," asparagus is an effective kidney diuretic. The asparagine breaks up oxalic and uric acid crystals that are in the kidneys and the muscles, and eliminates them through the urine.

Season: Spring.

Beans—Green (or yellow) snap beans are a popular addition to the garden that many people appreciate raw. I remember eating raw snap beans in my grandmother's garden during the summer as a kid, and never thinking that they would have been better cooked. They are best eaten straight from the garden, but if you buy them at the store, look for firm, long, slender, fresh, and vibrantly colored beans. Beans are believed to be native to the Mediterranean.

Health Benefits: Beans are rich in potassium, calcium, and minerals.

Season: Summer

Beet—Beets are a common root vegetable that can be appreciated raw. They are particularly colorful, and can be used as a decorative element in your raw creations. Grated beets can be added to salads. When buying beets, look for healthy, firm, wrinkle-free ones. Beets can keep a long time, as most root vegetables do. Beet juice can be used in combination with other green juices.

Health benefits: Beets are rich in iron, and are good for building healthy blood.

Season: Fall and Winter

Broccoli—Broccoli is related to cauliflower, and is commonly eaten steamed by many people concerned with their health and weight. Raw broccoli is good, and can be used in salads, or with dips and guacamole. Many people complain that they cannot eat broccoli raw without suffering from indigestion and gas. I understand that many are not used to eating fibrous foods, and therefore I would recommend eating smaller quantities, and chewing very thoroughly, rather than cooking it. When your digestion improves with time, you may find that you can eat raw broccoli in quantity, and without any discomfort.

Health benefits: Broccoli is rich in calcium, and is recommended for those suffering from acidosis conditions.

Season: Fall and Winter

Cabbage—Cabbage is native to Asia and is one of the most ancient vegetables. The philosopher Pythagoras (a vegetarian) liked cabbage so much that he wrote a whole book on it. Commonly used in both the cooked and raw form, most people know cabbage creates a horrible smell when it is cooked. Why have this problem when you can eat it raw and enjoy it even more? Raw cabbage does not cause the digestive inconvenience of cooked cabbage.

There are basically two varieties of cabbage: green and red. I like to call the red cabbage "purple," and the green cabbage "white," because it corresponds more to reality. There are many other varieties, which will not be discussed here. Cabbage is easily available organic, so there is no reason to buy commercial cabbage, as the organic type tastes much better Cabbage can be eaten chopped or grated, and mixed with a raw mayonnaise for a raw coleslaw, or added to salads. You can take a perfect leaf of purple cabbage, and fill it with guacamole, or nut pâté, and have a raw burrito!

Fermenting shredded cabbage in a container placed in a warm spot for a week makes sauerkraut. Most brands of sauerkraut in the store are cooked and contain added table salt. You can find raw sauerkraut in some health food stores. Raw, salt-free sauerkraut is useful for restoring the good bacteria that forms the bacterial flora in the digestive tract.

Health benefits: Cabbage is rich in minerals, and some even contain more calcium than broccoli. It is one of the least expensive, nutrient-rich foods. Cabbage is good for stimulating the immune system, healing ulcers, killing harmful bacteria, and clearing the complexion. Cabbage juice is particularly helpful for people suffering from ulcers and digestive problems.

Season: All Year

Carrot—Carrots are a popular raw vegetable, but ae highly hybridized, with a sugar content that is much higher than would exist in carrots growing in the wild. The wild carrot is not even orange, but purple. Drinking a lot of carrot juice will raise your blood sugar very fast, with the corresponding drop afterwards. Many health food folks drink a lot of carrot juice, thinking that they are doing something good for their body. While it is definitely better and more nutritious than drinking soda or artificial juices, it is not a good practice. The occasional raw carrot or carrot juice is fine, but the habit of drinking large quantities of carrot juice should be avoided.

Health benefits: Carrots are abundant in beta-carotene, which is a powerful antioxidant. As you may know, antioxidants are substances, such as vitamins E and C, which can prevent cell damage caused by oxidation.

Season: All Year.

Cauliflower—The cauliflower is related to the cabbage and, like broccoli, is another popular vegetable member of the cruciferous family. The cruciferous family of plants also comprises broccoli, cabbage, kale, and Brussels sprouts. Cauliflower can be chopped in salads, or used to dip in pates and guacamole.

Health benefits: Cauliflower is rich in calcium, boron, iron, and other minerals. Like all cruciferous vegetables, it is reputed to have cancer-fighting nutrients in the form of antioxidants. It is rich in sulfur, and therefore should not be eaten in very large quantities, or else it may cause slight indigestion.

Season: Fall and Winter

Celeriac—This is a special variety of celery, cultivated for its base rather than its branches. Many people think it is the weirdest-looking vegetable. It looks like an irregular root, the size of a big turnip, with many smaller roots extending from its base. It can be as small as a tomato, or as large as a cantaloupe.

Celeriac is very popular in some parts of Europe, but has never been very popular in North America, although we start to see it more and more in the health food stores and produce markets. It tastes like celery with a little bit of parsley. It is as hard as a carrot but not as juicy, and needs to be peeled before using. It can be grated and added to salads, or cut into sticks and dipped in guacamole or other raw dips. Also, I have created a delicious soup with it **(See the book "Easy Gourmet Raw Food Cuisine).**

Health benefits: Celeriac is rich in calcium, and has been known as a diuretic food.

Season: Fall and Winter

Celery—Celery is the favorite food of the gorilla, and could potentially become one of your favorites too. The wild variety of celery that the gorillas feed on is more bitter than the cultivated variety, which is sweet and tender. Organically grown celery should be the only type you purchase. This is because celery ranks high on the list of chemically farmed foods.

Health benefits: The major nutritional value of celery is its high organic sodium content. Eating celery on a regular basis, while following a mostly salt-free diet, will help you stay balanced, as sodium is a much-needed mineral. Eating celery or drinking celery juice during the hot months of the year will help hydrate your body. Besides sodium, celery is very rich in calcium and other alkaline minerals. It is helpful for persons suffering from indigestion and acidosis conditions.

Season: All year

Chard—Chard is a vegetable eaten for its green leaves that are rich in chlorophyll. It is native to China. When the plant is young, it is particularly good. It has a very salty taste and is excellent mixed with raw salads, or juiced with other vegetables. I have found that homegrown chard is superior to store- bought chard, the latter often being bitter.

Health benefits: Chard is rich in calcium, sulfur, potassium, and iron. It also contains moderate amounts of oxalic acids, but not enough to cause problems.

Season: Fall and Winter

Collards—Collards, or "collard greens," are like large, firm lettuce leaves. They are a member of the cabbage family, and are native to the Eastern Mediterranean countries. They can be grown easily in both hot and cold climates. In the United States, they are eaten mainly in the southern states, but their popularity is growing elsewhere.

Health benefits: Collards are a wonderful source of minerals, much richer than cabbage or spinach. They can be added to salads, juiced, or used as a wrap in place of tortillas for raw burritos.

Season: Fall, Winter and Spring.

Corn—Corn is actually a grain, but eaten fresh as a vegetable. In North America, fresh corn is synonymous with the abundance of late summer and fall, and festive summer parties. Generally it is eaten boiled and slathered with butter and salt. Most people do not know that corn can be eaten raw, and that it may even taste better that way. To enjoy raw fresh corn, make sure that it is freshly picked. After corn has been removed from the stalks, its sugar content quickly begins to turn into starch. This is why you will only appreciate raw corn if it has been picked the same day you eat it.

All you have to do to eat raw corn is peel and dive your teeth into it, or slice the corn kernels off of the ear with a knife. No time is wasted in boiling it, or in messing up the kitchen with melting butter. You can also scrape the kernels off with a knife, and add these to salads, salsas, and soups.

Health benefits: Corn is rich in many vitamins, but does not contain a lot of minerals. Therefore it is good to eat when it is in season, but definitely not as a staple in the diet.

Season: Summer

Dandelion—This is a plant that grows wild everywhere, and that you should get better acquainted with. Many people desperately try to prevent it from invading their yards, not knowing what a valuable plant it is. If you think dandelion is too bitter, try eating the young leaves, instead of the large older ones. You can pick wild dandelion, or buy the cultivated variety, which has a similar taste and nutritional value to the wild variety.

Health benefits: Dandelion has more beta-carotene, calcium and many more minerals than most cultivated vegetables. It is known to be a liver cleanser, and to neutralize acids in the body. If you have the right type of juicer, you can use dandelion juice in conjunction with other green juices and gain tremendous benefit out of it.

Season: Spring in northern countries, all year in southern countries.

Green onion—See Onion.

Jicama—The jicama (pronounce Hi-ca-ma) plant is very popular in Mexico, where it originates. It is used for its big, potato-like root. Although most people enjoy it cooked, you can also eat it raw. After peeling, you can slice it multiple ways and use it like potato chips to eat with guacamole or other dips. Jicama is crunchy, juicy, a little sweet, and not as starchy as a potato. For a delicious Jicama Salad, see **the book "Easy Gourmet Raw Food Cuisine".**

Health benefits: Jicama is abundant in fiber, potassium, iron, calcium, and vitamin A, B complex, and C.

Season: All year

Kale—Due to its nutritional value, kale is one of the most important of all the leafy green vegetables. Kale is native to the eastern Mediterranean region. It comes in many varieties, of which most are very tasty. My personal favorite is called "dinosaur" or "lacinto" kale. Many people think you have to steam kale, and that it is too coarse to be eaten raw with delight. But if you chew it long enough, and start with small quantities, you will soon be able to eat raw kale without trouble. You may also juice it, or blend it in raw soups to get all the nutritional benefits of this wonderful green vegetable.

Health benefits: Kale is rich in calcium, iron, sodium, and other important minerals, as well as vitamins. Just 100 grams of kale contains over 135 mg. of calcium.

Season: Fall and Winter

Lettuce & Salad Greens—Lettuce is the most common vegetable, and often the most common salad item. It is said to be native to Asia and Africa. There are many varieties of lettuce from which to choose. These include Boston lettuce, leaf or red leaf, Romaine, and the less exciting iceberg lettuce. In this category we also include the other salad greens, such as arugula, pepper grass, escarole, chicory, watercress, and all the other greens. Select lettuce heads and salad greens that are fresh, crisp, and not wilted. If they are wilted, as they often may be during the winter months, you can discard the outer leaves and eat the fresher and more nutritious inside leaves. As a general rule, the more vibrant its color, the more nutritious the lettuce will be. Rather than eat the same type of lettuce all the time, experiment with the various types of lettuce and salad greens. My personal favorites are Romaine lettuce and arugula. I use arugula as a flavoring in salads and other dishes.

Health benefits: Lettuce and salad greens are an important source of minerals. The milky juice found in the stems of some types of lettuce have sedative properties, and may make you sleepy. So if you need a good night's sleep, have a salad with lots of romaine lettuce and salad greens. Lettuce is also rich in vitamin E, which is a key element in the reproductive process. In other words: salads are good for sex.

Season: Lettuce and salad greens are abundant in Summer and early Fall.

Mushrooms—Mushrooms are an edible fungi, which are simple plants that live in moist and cool places. Mushrooms lack the chlorophyll needed to photosynthesize nutrients from the sun, and therefore have to receive their nourishment from other organic matter. There are thousands of varieties of mushrooms growing in the wild—including some that are very poisonous. I would recommend eating the cultivated varieties, and forget about foraging for mushrooms in the wild unless you are absolutely positive that you know what you are doing. Some poisonous types are capable of killing you within hours after eating them.

Popular varieties of mushrooms (besides the common white mushroom) include portobello and shiitake, which are very good in recipes. The portobello mushroom is my favorite, being big and meaty. It can be served in salads, marinated, or used in "Portobello Supreme" **(See the book "Easy Gourmet Raw Food Cuisine").**

Health benefits: Mushrooms are rich in zinc and a few other minerals, including germanium which helps counteract pollution.

Season: All year

Mustard Greens—Mustard greens originate from Asia, where they have been grown for thousands of years. In the United States they are popular in the South but

71

like collard greens, the popularity of mustard greens is spreading. Generally these greens are cooked, but as with most vegetables, they can be appreciated raw in salads. Mustard greens are quite strong, but can be eaten in small quantities, mixed with milder vegetables.

Health Benefits: Mustard greens are rich in calcium and other minerals. They help to alkalinize the body, as well as assist it in ridding itself of toxic substances.

Season: Fall, Winter and Spring.

Onion—As Sanskrit and Hebrew literature indicate, onions have been cultivated longer than most vegetables. Onions are often used for flavoring and can be added to many dishes. Green onions are the green leaves that sprout from the onion bulb, and are sold as a different vegetable. Shallots are used the same way as onions in small quantities as a flavoring.

Health benefits: Onions are a wonderful food that possess antibiotic-like qualities, are a diuretic, blood pressure regulator, and antiseptic. Onions can be helpful in ridding the intestinal tract of parasites.

Season: All year

Radish—Radishes are strong flavored bulbous roots. They are native to China, and have been eaten in Egypt since the beginning of their civilization. There are a few varieties available, the most common being the small red radish. Bigger, black radishes are also cultivated and are a variety that keeps well during the winter. Radishes are commonly used in salads, but can also be eaten on their own.

Health Benefits: Radishes are rich in sulfur, which is an important element for skin beauty.

Season: Sprint, Summer and Winter (for Winter varieties).

Shallots—See Onion.

Spinach—Spinach originally comes from northern Asia, and is now one of the most cultivated green vegetables. There are many varieties which are all excellent. Many people do not like spinach because of the way it is traditionally prepared: cooked. Raw spinach is much more pleasing to the palate. You can juice it along with other vegetables for a healthy drink. It is also good chopped and added to many different dishes, and blended into raw soups.

Health benefits: Raw spinach is an excellent food for detoxifying the digestive tract and restoring pH balance. It is rich in minerals, especially iron (as Popeye knew—although the cooked, canned spinach Popeye was eating would not be recommended). Spinach also contains a notable quantity of oxalic acid, and therefore it would be a good idea not to eat too much of it, or eat it too often, since oxalic acid is reputed to hinder the absorption of calcium. However, many people eat spinach every day, and do not seem to suffer any negative effects from this.

Season: Summer and Fall.

Sprouts—When you soak any seed in water, it sprouts, releasing all of its stored nutrients, enzymes, and life-giving potential. When this was discovered, the practice of sprouting the seeds of alfalfa, buckwheat, sunflower and other seeds in order to eat the young plant they produced became popular. Ann Wigmore was one of the first people to promote the health benefits of sprouts. Nowadays, you can find sprouts in most every food market, and as part of the food offerings in many restaurants.

Sprouts are useful for many reasons. Sprouts are vegetables that with a little time and investment are easy to grow. Sprouts are ready to be harvested within a week. With the knowledge of sprouting, good nutrition is now possible in the most extreme situations such as cold winters, food supply exhaustion, long trips in the woods or the ocean, etc. You can eat sprouts on their own, or mix them with salads.

Health benefits: During sprouting, the vitamin and enzyme content of seeds increases dramatically, while starch is being converted into simple sugars, and all the other nutrients become more assimilable. The fresher the sprouts are, the more nutritious they will be. So it is better to grow your own sprouts, which is quite easy to do. There are many books on the subject that can guide you in the process of sprouting a variety of seeds.

The best sprouts are those which turn into little green plants, such as sunflower greens and buckwheat greens. Some sprouts, such as bean and grain sprouts, will still contain high amounts of raw starch, which is not totally transformed into simple sugar. Because raw starch is difficult to digest, it is better to eat these starchy sprouts sparingly. The best varieties include clover, buckwheat greens, sunflower greens, fenugreek, mustard, and radish. The starchy sprouts include: wheat berries, mung beans, and chickpeas.

Season: All year Sprouts may be grown at any time of the year in any climate, as long as a warm place with sonic light is provided.

Sweet Potato & Yam—These tubers, although they are not related, have similar characteristics. The typical white potato is not used in the raw food cuisine, due to the fact that it has a high starch content. But sweet potatoes and yams are closer to their wild ancestors, and are a staple item in many countries of the world. They may be eaten raw, grated in salads, or sliced as a dipping ingredient with guacamole or nut pâtés. Although you might think that raw sweet potatoes are not edible, you should try them at least once. Many raw-foodists occasionally enjoy the taste of raw sweet potatoes and yams. The sweet potato is native to the southern United States, while the yam is native to West Africa and Asia.

Health benefits: Sweet potatoes and yams are highly nutritious, and very alkaline when eaten raw. They contain a high amount of beta-carotene, and other important nutrients.

Season: Fall and Winter

Chapter 8
NUTS & SEEDS

Nuts and Seeds are a concentrated source of energy. While their use in the typical diet is often limited to snacks in a roasted and salted form, you will realize that nuts have a much more important role in the raw food cuisine. Nuts and seeds are rich in minerals, trace minerals, and essential fatty acids. Most people are deficient in essential fatty acids, because the majority of the fat they eat is cooked. Heated fat, such as fried oil, is carcinogenic and simply not good for the body.

Ideally, nuts and seeds should be bought raw and organically grown. Nuts in the shell and whole seeds are more superior than shelled nuts and refined seeds. In recipes we prefer to use shelled nuts to save time. To make them easier to digest, nuts and seeds can be soaked in water for a few hours.

Nuts and seeds may be used in various ways. They can be eaten on their own (ideally with green vegetables) as a snack. They can be added to salads, turned into milks and pâtés, added to smoothies, and used in sauces and dips. Since nuts are acid-forming, they should always be eaten with green vegetables, which are extremely alkaline.

ABOUT THE SOAKING OF NUTS AND SEEDS

Many recipes in this book call for soaked nuts and seeds. We soak the nuts because it makes them easier to digest. Also, it is sometimes necessary to achieve the desired consistency in the recipes. I recommend that you soak your nuts and seeds the night before using them. Place a little more than half of the quantity you intend to use the next day into a bowl, and cover with purified water. They will almost double in volume. Do that before you go to sleep. The next morning, strain the water, rinse the nuts or seeds, and place in the refrigerator until you are ready to use them. You may also soak them in the morning for use in the evening. Plan on soaking them for 6-12 hours. If you do not have that amount of time, try to soak them for at least a few hours anyway.

NUTS

Almond—Most almonds available in North America are grown in California. Almonds are one of the sweetest of all nuts, and a popular ingredient in the raw food cuisine. Almonds should be bought organic because non-organic almonds are likely to contain heavy doses of toxic chemicals. Almonds can be used to make delicious milks, nut butters, pâtés, sauces, and raw candies. The almond tree is native to North Africa, West Asia, and the Mediterranean.

Health benefits: Almonds are rich in calcium, as well as many other minerals which are useful for building up a body which is underweight. For best assimilation, almonds should be soaked and masticated thoroughly.

Season: Fall and Winter.

Brazil Nut—Brazil nuts grow wild in the jungles of South America. Even today, the Brazil nuts you purchase are likely to come from wild trees, which are huge evergreens whose trunks may grow up to six feet in diameter, and reach the immense height of 150 feet! These nuts have a pleasing rich flavor, and are one of the richest nuts in fat. It is preferable to buy them in the shell, as shelled Brazil nuts have been boiled to release them from their shell.

Health benefits: With their high fat content, Brazil nuts are useful for those doing hard physical work, or for individuals needing to gain some weight. They are acid-forming, and should always be eaten with green vegetables.

Season: Fall and Winter.

Cashew—Cashews are a seed that grow at the base of the fruit called the "cashew apple." The fruit contains a sweet liquid, and is used as a drink in the tropical countries where the cashew tree grows, mainly in Central America. The nut has to be slightly heated in order to get rid of some acids. I have heard that it is also possible to sun-dry the nut to achieve the same result. There is a lot of controversy concerning the cashew nut. Many believe that it is not a living food, since it has to be heated before consumption. If they sprout, then they can be considered alive (raw), otherwise they are dead (cooked). Cashews can be turned into delicious nut milks **(See the book "Easy Gourmet Raw Food Cuisine"),** blended into smoothies, dressings, scattered into salads, made into nut butters or pâtés, or eaten on their own.

Health benefits: Cashews are rich in calories and therefore useful for the very active person, or the individual who needs to gain weight.

Season: All year

Coconut—The coconut is the queen of all nuts. I say this because coconuts provide both solid and liquid food. It is a staple in the diets of the tropical countries where it grows. To get the nuts, someone has to climb to the top of the palm trees on which the coconuts grow. This is how coconuts have always been harvested, including those in your local supermarket. They are believed to be native from Polynesia, Malaysia, and southern Asia.

As coconuts ripen, the meat inside of them becomes firm. The brown coconuts sold in supermarkets are the mature" coconuts, with a hard meat and sweet milk. When picked before that stage, the meat inside of the coconut is soft, and can be eaten with a spoon. These are then called "young coconuts," or "spoon-meat coconuts" and are white-husked. They are our favorite, and can be obtained at many Asian Markets. Many health food stores are beginning to carry young coconuts and, even if they do not, they may be willing to order some for you at the cost of about $1 to $1.50 each. Young coconut meat can be eaten plain, or blended into smoothies, soups, or dressings.

Homemade, freshly shredded coconut may be obtained by processing the meat of mature coconuts in a food processor or Champion Juicer. It can be used in the preparation of living desserts. Blending the hard coconut meat with its water, and filtering out bits of coconuts by pouring through a strainer makes coconut milk. It can be used as any other nut milk. Coconut water is the liquid inside of the coconut. It can be consumed as it is, or blended into soups or smoothies. Coconut cream is made by juicing the hard coconut meat with a Champion, Green Power, or Green Life juicer (or any other mastication or twin-gear juicer). It can be used in place of milk cream. Coconut butter is simply coconut oil. Since coconut oil is solid at room temperature, it has the appearance of butter. Coconut butter may be used in place of regular butter—as a transition food—and also used in place of other types of oils. It is high in saturated fat, which may be of concern to people with cholesterol problems. But it should be noted that there is no proof that saturated fat coming from a natural source, such as coconuts, cause any of the same health challenges as saturated fat coming from animal sources. Many nations eat plenty of coconut everyday, and do not suffer from the cholesterol problems seen in countries where saturated fat from animals is consumed.

In my opinion, one of the reasons why coconuts are the best nuts is that they are fresh. Many nuts available in stores have been dried, heated, or salted. With coconuts, you know that they are still alive and unprocessed.

Health Benefits: Coconut water is rich in calcium and trace minerals, and can be used to remineralize the body and provide sustenance with its sweet water. Coconut meat is rich in saturated fatty acids, and is a perfect body building food.

Season: All year

Hazelnut or Filbert—Different varieties of these nuts are native to North America, Asia, and Europe. They still grow wild across the northern part of the United States, and are grown commercially in the states of Oregon and Washington.

Health benefits: When eaten in combination with green vegetables, they form a wonderful body building food. They are also rich in calcium and trace minerals.

Season: Fall and Winter

Macadamia Nut—Macadamias are often the favorite nut of raw vegans due to their high fat content, brittle crunchiness, and incredible flavor. They originate from Australia, where they still grow wild. It has only been 150 years since farmers began cultivating these delicious nuts. They are usually more expensive than other nuts, and considered a delicacy by many people. But, because many farmers in California and Hawaii are now growing them, macadamia nuts have become less expensive, and more popular. The nuts are contained within a very hard shell, which resists most nutcrackers. There is one nutcracker that will do the trick, called the Krakanut. If you buy nuts in the shell it is a necessary investment! You can also buy them shelled, but as with all nuts, it is better to buy them in the shell, as they will be fresher.

Health benefits: Macadamia nuts are rich in all of the essential fatty acids, offer a better balance of these acids than most nuts, and contain a larger amount of the Omega-3 fatty acid, which is the one that we usually need more of. They also contain plenty of trace minerals, and form a great bodybuilding meal when they are eaten in combination with green vegetables.

Season: Fall and Winter

Pecan—Pecans are native to North America, and still grow wild in some areas of the country. The trees are very long-lived, and some of them are thought to be over a thousand years old. Pecans have a fine flavor and high mineral content, which makes them appropriate in the creation of living desserts.

Pecans are also delicious when added to salads, or simply eaten alone.

Health benefits: Pecans are one of the richest plant sources of vitamin B6, which plays an important role in the nervous system. Their mineral and fatty acid profile also makes them good for those needing to rejuvenate their heart.

Season: Fall.

Pine Nut—Pine nuts are the seeds from the cones of certain species of pine trees. They have the most delicate, buttery taste of all the nuts, and are used in many gourmet raw vegan meals. For added taste and nutrition, you can sprinkle them onto your salads, dips, and sauces.

Health benefits: Pine nuts are rich in quality proteins, and many trace minerals.

Season: Fall.

Pistachio—Pistachios are delicious nuts, which are appreciated in Middle Eastern countries. In America, salted pistachios are sold at sporting events. This nut has a unique and delicate flavor. We like to add them to salads.

Most pistachios found in markets, and even health food stores, are roasted, dyed, salted, or processed through other means. There are a few places that sell raw, natural pistachios—and they are listed at the end of this book.

Health benefits: Pistachios contain little fiber, and are therefore easy to digest and assimilate. Raw pistachios are useful in purifying the blood, and in helping to maintain a healthy liver and kidneys.

Season: Fall and Winter

Walnut—Walnuts are one of the most popular nuts in North America. Many varieties of walnuts, including the black walnut, are indigenous to North America. Some varieties of walnuts include: Chinese walnut, Japanese walnut, white walnut (also called butternut) and English walnut.

Due to their high oil content, walnuts tend to go rancid quickly, and should be bought in the shell whenever possible. They should be stored in a cool, dry place. Walnuts may be added to salads, or used in nut pâtés, turned into milks, and used in raw desserts. I like to use walnuts as a base for raw pie crusts.

Health benefits: Walnuts are a good food for improving the metabolism, and for strengthening the kidneys and lungs. Black walnuts are an old proven remedy for ridding the intestines of parasites.

Season: Fall and Winter

SEEDS

Flax—Flax is a plant grown for its fiber, which is used to make cloth (linen). The seeds of the plant are also cultivated, as they are highly nutritious. The tiny, shiny, dark brown or golden seeds may be ground and added to smoothies and dressings. They have to be ground beforehand, in order to be assimilable by the body. The seeds can be used to make flax crackers (**see the book "Easy Gourmet Raw Food Cuisine"**). We use their oil in salad dressings, soups, and other dishes to enhance flavor, texture, and to add essential fatty acids.

Health benefits: Flax seeds (and flax seed oil) are rich in Omega-3, an essential fatty acid (EFA). This EFA helps people with heart problems, and is also an important nutrient for the brain. Flax seeds also contain plant hormones, and are high in potassium, magnesium, calcium, iron, lecithin, and vitamin E.

Season: All year

Pumpkin—Pumpkin seeds are very tasty and nutritious, and can be used in salads, nut pâtés, and soups. Also, they may be eaten as a snack on their own, or ground and added to salads. It is better to grind pumpkin seeds before adding them to salads, in order to get the maximum nutrition available.

Health benefits: Pumpkin seeds are rich in zinc and magnesium, which make them a most nourishing food for the sexually active male, as these minerals are used in the production of semen.

Season: Late summer and Fall

Sesame—Sesame is another popular seed. It is commonly consumed in the form of tahini, which is nothing more than butter made out of hulled sesame seeds. Unhulled seeds have a stronger taste than hulled seeds and are alkalizing. Hulled seeds are used mainly in the preparation of tahini. Tahini made out of unhulled sesame seeds is usually called "sesame butter." Sesame seeds come from a tall herb, and are grown in Africa and Asia. Tahini is a common food in Middle Eastern countries, while sesame oil is widely used in Chinese cooking. Whole, raw sesame seeds are great to use in raw candy, which can be made by mixing sesame seeds with blended dates, then rolling small balls of this into shredded coconuts and chopped nuts.

Health Benefits: Unhulled sesame seeds are rich in calcium, and may be ground and mixed with smoothies, or added to salads in order to add minerals to the diet. Sesame seeds are high in Vitamin E, which strengthens the heart and nerves.

Season: September through April

Sunflower—Sunflower seeds grow on a majestic plant that is native to the Americas and that has been made famous by Vincent Van Gogh, who was fascinated by the beauty of the sunflowers in the fields of the French countryside. They may be used in nut pâtés, turned into delicious milks, or enjoyed as a snack on their own. The unhulled seeds may be sprouted and enjoyed as a nutritious green vegetable, when the plant has grown a couple inches tall with little green leaves. At that stage they are full of vitality and sun energy.

Health Benefits: The sunflower seed is a rich source of vitamin D, B complex, E, and K. They are also a rich source of high-quality protein.

Season: Fall and Winter

Chapter 9

SPICES, CONDIMENTS & SPECIAL INGREDIENTS

In this section we will discuss the spices, condiments and special ingredients that are used in the raw food cuisine. Some of these ingredients may already be familiar to you, and others may not. You do not need all these ingredients to make great food, but I use some of them quite often as you will discover by making the recipes in this book. Many of these ingredients may be bought at your local health food store.

Condiments can really make the raw food cuisine sparkle. You may choose not to use them, if you prefer the taste of unseasoned food. Some purists may object to some of these items, saying that they are not "living" or raw. My response to this is, correct—some of these condiments are other than living. But they are used only for flavor, and in such small quantities that I cannot see how they could reduce the vitality otherwise attained through following a raw food diet.

HERBS AND SPICES

Remember that most spices and dried herbs are irradiated, so look for non-irradiated spices and always seek out those that have been grown organically. Many of these herbs can be obtained fresh at the market or from your garden.

If you have access to fresh herbs, I recommend using them over dried herbs. If you substitute fresh herbs for dried herbs in one of the recipes, use 3-4 times as much of the fresh as the stated quantity of dried herbs listed in the recipe. However, I sometimes deliberately use dried herbs even though the fresh ones are obtainable. For example, the taste of powdered garlic is different than the taste of fresh garlic. Sometimes I like to use powdered garlic to achieve a particular taste in a recipe.

Basil—Also called sweet basil, it is native to India and Iran. There exist a few varieties including small-leaf common basil, larger leaf Italian basil, purple basil, lemon basil, and the large lettuce-leaf basil. It most often associated with Italian cuisine. It is excellent with tomatoes and in salads.

Cardamom—A spice consisting of the whole or ground dried fruit, or seeds, of a plant member from the ginger family, native to the moist forests of southern India. It a popular seasoning in Oriental dishes, and commonly used in the preparation of Chai, an Indian spiced tea.

Cayenne—Dried hot powder made out of the cayenne pepper, and used to spice a variety of dishes. Cayenne pepper is native to the warmer regions of Asia and America, and is now cultivated in all parts of the world. It is very spicy and should be used carefully.

Chili powder—A blend of spices, often containing cayenne pepper, oregano, paprika, cumin, and garlic.

Chives—A plant related to the onion, chives are native to Asia and Europe, and are grown for their tubular leaves which grow in clumps. They may be used to flavor soups and salads.

Cinnamon—A powder made out of the inner bark of a tree, excellent for flavoring anything sweet. It is one of the oldest known spices and is native to Sri Lanka. The spice is light brown in color and has a delicate fragrant aroma and warm sweet flavor. Cinnamon was once more valuable than gold. In the United States it is especially popular in baked goods. It can be purchased whole or in a powder form.

Cilantro—Native to the Mediterranean and Middle East regions, cilantro is cultivated in Europe, Morocco, and the United States for its seeds, which are turned into a powder called coriander. The fresh leaves are used in Latin American, Indian, and Chinese dishes. It can be added to all sorts of dishes. If fresh cilantro is not available, it can be replaced by fresh parsley.

Clove—The word "clove" comes from the French "clou," meaning "nail." The clove tree is believed to have originated in China. The spice comes from the buds of a tree, which are sun-dried and turned into a powder, or sold whole. Cloves are highly aromatic, and used to spice pies and nut milks.

Cumin—Cumin is native to the Mediterranean region, and also cultivated in India, China, and Mexico for its seeds, which are turned into a powder and used to flavor a variety of dishes. Cumin is an excellent spice to use in guacamole.

Curry—A combination of spices. The basic ingredients in curry powder are turmeric (which gives the yellow color), cumin, coriander, and red (or cayenne) pepper. It is popular in Indian cuisine.

Dill—A member of the parsley family, dill is native to Mediterranean countries and southeastern Europe, and now widely cultivated in Europe, India, and North America. It can be used for its leaves or seeds, which are very aromatic. It is very popular in Persian cuisine.

Fennel—Fennel is a plant that has a licorice flavor, and can be used as a flavoring. It originates from southern Europe, and now grows wild in various locations, including the United States. It is sold in a few stores as a vegetable, which can be used for its aromatic bulb, stalks, and leaves. Good in salads.

Garlic—Garlic is a bulb native to the Mediterranean regions of Africa and Europe. The bulb separates into segments that are called cloves. Garlic is considered one of the most important spices in healthy cuisine and we use it to flavor many dishes. Garlic keeps a long time when it is stored in a cool dry place. One thing you can do with the cloves is plant them in a pot, and use the flavorsome garlic greens in salads, soups, and as garnishes. Garlic is one of the best antibacterial and antiseptic plants. Eat raw garlic to rid the intestines of parasites. It can be used to boost the immune system, purify the bloodstream, and also regulate the action of the liver and kidneys.

Garlic powder—Powder made out of dried garlic cloves. Garlic powder has a slightly different and mellower flavor than fresh garlic.

Ginger—The ginger plant is believed to be native to southeastern Asia. It is grown for its aromatic underground stem, part of the plant which is called a "rhizome." People call it "ginger root," although it is not an accurate designation. It is used as a spice, flavoring, food, and medicine. Its use in India and China has been known from ancient times. Ginger can be used fresh or in a powder form. It is wonderful when used to enhance the flavor of many raw dishes, dressings, and juices.

Italian herb mix—A mix of dried herbs, usually consisting of oregano, marjoram, thyme, rosemary, basil, and sage. Usually sold under the name "Italian Seasoning."

Marjoram—A member of the mint family, used for its leaves and flowering tops, either fresh or dried, to flavor many foods. Marjoram is native to the Mediterranean. It tastes similar to oregano.

Mint—The mint plant, which is used for its aromatic leaves, is native to the Near East, and now grows all over the world. Mint leaves are refreshing, and can be used fresh or dried. I like to add mint to fruit salads and other desserts.

Mustard—Mustard plants and seeds are mentioned frequently in Greek and Roman writings and in the Bible. As a condiment, mustard is sold in three forms: as seeds, as dry powder, and as a paste that is blended with other spices, salt, and vinegar. I have been able to find a mustard condiment in some health food stores, made with mustard seeds, apple cider vinegar, and sea salt. It is made by a company called "Eden" and is much healthier than regular mustard.

Nutmeg—Nutmeg is native to Indonesia. It is the dried seed of a fruit, used as an aromatic spice. It can be bought whole or ground. It has a sweet, spicy and sharp flavor, and is usually used to flavor desserts.

Oregano—Another herb member of the mint family, widely used to season many foods. Oregano can be used fresh or dried. It is native to the Mediterranean countries and western Asia. It is popular as a seasoning in pizza.

Paprika—A spice made from the pods of a chili pepper plant native to tropical areas of the Western Hemisphere, including Mexico, Central America, South America, and the West Indies. The pods are then dried and ground to produce paprika. It is frequently used in the cooking of Spain, Mexico, and Hungary.

Parsley—Parsley is considered to be an herb, and is often used for decorative purposes. Parsley may be added to salads, blended into soups, and juiced. The most common variety of parsley is called "curly" parsley. Italian parsley is another variety with flat, long leaves. Both are good. Parsley is believed to be native from Turkey, where it still grows wild.

Parsley flakes—Parsley in a dried form.

Pizza seasonings—A mix of herbs, usually consisting of oregano, marjoram, basil, red bell pepper, and powdered garlic.

Pepper—A pungent spice made from the berries of a plant. One of the earliest spices known to humans, and widely used in the world today. Comes in many varieties, including black and white pepper.

Rosemary—Leaves of a shrub, and a member of the mint family. Can be used fresh or dried. The leaves have a very powerful taste, so they must be used sparingly. Rosemary is native to the Mediterranean region, and has been naturalized throughout Europe and temperate America.

Sage—An aromatic herb native to the Mediterranean region, cultivated for its leaves, which are used fresh or dried. Has a powerful flavor.

Thyme—A pungent herb member of the mint family, used for its leaves and flowering tops, fresh or dried. Thyme is native to southern Europe, the Mediterranean region, Asia Minor, and Central Asia, and is also cultivated in North America. Dried thyme leaves are greenish-brown in color, and have a fragrant odor when crushed.

Turmeric—Turmeric is the dried root of a plant related to ginger Sold in a ground form, it is widely used in Indian curries. It will "color" any foods to which it is added a warm yellow-orange.

OTHER SPECIAL INGREDIENTS
and CONDIMENTS

You might not be familiar with some of the ingredients used in this book. Do not panic because almost all of these ingredients may be bought in your local health food store.

Almond butter—Almond butter is made out of ground almonds, and is considered to be a living food when bought "raw." It is sweet, creamy, and very satisfying. It is good spread on apple slices, and may be used in many recipes.

Apple cider vinegar—A vinegar made out of aged apple cider Buy it raw and unpasteurized. It is wonderful in salad dressings.

Bragg's Liquid Aminos—This liquid seasoning, commonly called "Bragg's," is very popular in raw food circles. It is made from soybeans and has not been fermented. I choose not to use it in the recipes of this book, because many people question its "rawness." However, if it agrees with you, you may use it in place of Nama Shoyu, or tamari sauce, in the recipes of this book.

Carob powder—Carob powder is made from the dried carob pod, and is used as a chocolate replacement. While chocolate is a stimulant, carob helps calm the nerves.

Coconut water—The sweet, mineral-rich water found inside a coconut.

Dulse flakes—Dulse that has been dried and cut into tiny pieces. Dulse is a delicious type of seaweed. It can be found in most health food stores, or purchased through mail-order companies specializing in sea vegetables.

Flax seed oil—A very nutritious oil that is rich in essential fatty acids. Buy only if sold in glass bottles, and is labelled cold-pressed and organic. The oil then needs to be stored in a cool, dark place.

Fresh leaf herbs—Leaf herbs, such as dill, basil, mint, oregano, and thyme, are much more flavorsome when fresh. You may find fresh herbs at the health food stores, or grow them yourself. Add them to everything that you make which is not sweet.

Garlic-Chili flavored flax seed oil—A very tasty oil, flavored with garlic and chilis. It is made by an American company called Omega. But it can also be made at home by soaking a few garlic cloves and chili peppers in 2 cups of flax seed or olive oil.

Green olives—Green olives are often picked before maturity and pickled in a special solution that includes vinegar. Some olives are cured in water only.

Hemp seed oil—One of the most nutritious of all oils because it contains the perfect balance of essential fatty acids. Hemp seed oil has a pleasant, nutty flavor. It can be used with, or in place of, olive oil. It is now increasing in popularity, and is available cold-pressed in many health food stores.

Honey—Different types of honey are available, usually named after the flowers that fed the bees or after a town or region where the honey was gathered. There is wildflower honey, orange blossom, buckwheat, etc. Many varieties of honey sold on the market have been heated, which destroys the natural abundance of enzymes. The label "raw" does not mean anything as far as honey is concerned. It should mention "unheated." For those who object to honey for different reasons, you can replace honey in recipes with maple syrup or dates. For maple syrup, use twice the quantity. For dates, use 2-3 small dates to replace 1 Tbsp. of honey. You can soak the dates first in water for one or two hours to make them easier to mix with the other ingredients.

Jalapeno pepper—Pronounce, "Ha-la-pee-nio." A hot variety of pepper, used in small quantities to spice dishes, and very popular in Mexican cuisine. It is sold fresh. Available green and red.

Miso—Miso is a fermented product made out of soybeans. It is used in Asian cuisine, and comes in many flavors, my favorite being the mellow white miso. Buy it unpasteurized. You can find this in health food stores. It is not a totally "raw" product, since the soybeans are cooked. But after the long fermentation—a transformative enzymatic process—it is considered to be "living."

Nama Shoyu, or Tamari sauce—Nama Shoyu is a tasty soy sauce that is unpasteurized. While not being entirely raw (some cooked ingredients are used in the process), it can still be considered a living food, as it is rich in enzymes created during the fermentation process. If you do not find Nama Shoyu at your local health food store, you can buy "tamari sauce," which is a pasteurized version similar in taste. You may also order Nama Shoyu by mail order.

Olive oil—Purchase olive oil that is organic and cold pressed. The very best olive oil is "stone-pressed." Stone-pressed olive oil has been pressed using the ancient method of the Greeks. It has a very rich, fruity flavor, and is much more nutritious, due to the care taken at every step of the oil production process.

Pickled Ginger—Strips of peeled ginger that have been marinated in vinegar and sea salt. Can be found in most health food stores, near the sea vegetable section.

Sea salt—Sea salt should be bought totally unrefined. The best unrefined sea salt is sold under the name of "Celtic Sea Salt" in the health food stores. It often comes from France. But it can also be sold under other names. Good quality sea salt should still be slightly moist. You can buy it "coarse" or "fine." "Coarse" sea salt comes in bigger pieces, while "fine" sea salt looks more like regular table salt. I usually use the "coarse" variety, but most people prefer the "fine" variety for its ease of use.

Spirulina flakes—Spirulina is a form of edible algae usually sold as a food supplement, because of its extreme richness in protein, vitamins, minerals, and other nutrients. But it is really a food, and can be used as a regular item on the table. Spirulina is usually sold either in capsules, or in a powdered form. This type of Spirulina is not usually very tasty. But I have found a very good type of Spirulina, sold in flake form, with added lecithin. It is very tasty, and has a nice, salty quality.

Sun-dried olives—These are dried, black olives preserved in olive oil and sea salt. Sun-dried olives may be added to salads, or eaten on their own. To remove excess salt from the olives, you may soak them for a few days in water, changing the water twice a day.

Sun-dried tomatoes—Sun-dried tomatoes are often sold soaking in olive oil, but also plain in packages, or in bulk. We recommend the organic, sun-dried tomato halves, sold in bulk. Make sure they do not have any salt or chemical preservatives added. Even better, make your own sun-dried tomatoes during the tomato season, using a food dehydrator To use sun-dried tomatoes for a recipe, soak them first in water for at least one hour The longer they soak, the softer they will be. You can soak them up to 24 hours.

Tahini—This is a rich paste made out of hulled sesame seeds. Buy it raw and organic. Because of its great flavor, consistency, and nutritional value, tahini is commonly used in raw food cuisine.

Vanilla extract—Natural vanilla extract can be used to enhance the flavor of living desserts. Buy it without alcohol from the health food store.

Wild rice—Wild rice is not a true grain, but a seed. It is in fact not at all related to rice, but named that way because of its appearance. Wild rice grows in Canada and the northern United States, and is still harvested from the wild.

It is a really nutritious and hearty addition to raw food cuisine. Wild rice may be eaten raw, but has to be sprouted beforehand. Soak a cup or two of wild rice for 24 hours in ajar. Then drain the water, and rinse two times a day for the next two or three days until the rice is soft enough to eat. It usually takes 2 or 3 days of sprouting (plus one day of soaking). I like to soak wild rice in a large, glass container, and then place it in a large strainer, the same type that is used to drain pasta. It is then easy to run water over it twice a day. Place the strainer full of wild rice in a bowl, to avoid getting water everywhere. You may then make delicious salads with the wild rice, or add it to other dishes.

Young coconut meat—The tender flesh of a coconut that has been picked before maturity. You may find these young white "Thai" coconuts in many Asian markets.

Chapter 10
SEA VEGETABLES

Sea vegetables can help bring minerals to your diet. My friend, John Ferney, M.D., who is a big advocate of sea vegetables, says, "There are about one hundred minerals and trace minerals in the ocean. Human blood contains them all, and you must replace them on a regular basis. Seaweed is the way to bring these minerals into our diet, as they are integrated into the plant in a most assimilable form." Vegetables and fruits grown on large farms are becoming less reliable as good sources for minerals, as erosion and overfarming is creating poorer and poorer soil. Sea vegetables are wild plants that contain a bounty of minerals.

Arame—Similar to hijiki, but with a milder taste. It is harvested in Japan, and the Pacific North American coast. Arame has to be soaked 10 minutes before being used. It is a good source of iron, calcium, and iodine.

Dulse—This is our favorite sea vegetable. Dulse can be bought whole leaf or in flakes. We generally rinse whole leaf dulse for a few seconds, making it more tender and easier to cut. You can eat dulse on its own as a snack, or add it to salads, soups, and dips. It is an excellent source of iron and iodine. Seaweeds should be kept in a cool, dry place—preferably in a glass container.

Hijiki—This is a mild sea vegetable that has to be soaked for about 10 minutes before being used. It will quadruple in size as it soaks. It is rich in calcium and iron.

Kelp—The most common seaweed, kelp, is usually used in a powdered form. It is rich in minerals, and powdered kelp can be used in place of salt.

Nori—Nori is a popular seaweed that comes in thin sheets. These are used to make sushi or Nori rolls (**see Easy Gourmet Raw Food Cuisine**). The toasted Nori is greenish in appearance, while the sun-dried kind is black. Nori is rich in quality-protein, and in vitamins A, B1, and B3.

Wakame—A brown seaweed that grows in long, thin strips. Like hijiki, wakame should also be soaked before being used.

Chapter 11
THE EQUIPMENT

In the raw food cuisine, there are many things you will not need: stoves, microwaves, toasters, and other machines that heat food. Many of the tools you are familiar with, and may already have in your kitchen, are used in the preparation of raw foods.

COMMON TOOLS THAT ARE USED IN THE RAW FOOD CUISINE

Bowls • Cutting board • Funnel • Grater • Measuring cups • Pie server • Pie tins • Plates • Set of knives • Strainer • Vegetable peeler

Other tools, such as blenders, food processors, juicers, and dehydrators are also very useful. You will not need all of these tools in order to make most of the recipes in this book, but many of the tools, such as the Vita-Mix blender, are so versatile and useful that we use them on a daily basis. Remember that money invested in these tools is an investment in your health.

BLENDER—One of the most common and useful kitchen appliances is a blender. A blender liquefies foods, thus providing us with maximum nutrients, with less work needing to be done by the digestive system.

Your choice of a blender will determine the quality of your blended meals. Using low-end blenders for blending hard vegetables and leafy greens will be difficult, if not impossible—or, at least, very messy. You will need a good commercial type blender to do this. I have found the "Vita-Mix" to be the best blender. You will have to make sure that whatever model you purchase has a strong motor, and the capacity to blend a lot more than a typical blender. Try to get a heavy-duty blender that can hold twice as much as a regular blender.

VITA-MIX—The Vita-Mix (or a heavy-duty blender) is one of the most important tools you can use in your raw-vegan kitchen. So what is so great about this machine? Well, first of all, the Vita-Mix is more than a blender. True, it is a heavy-duty blender, but it does more than any typical, cheap blender. It can contain twice as much as a regular blender, and its heavy-duty motor can blend basically anything you put in there into a fine liquid. It is a powerful machine!

So what can you use the Vita-Mix for? Mostly, you will use it in the preparation of raw soups, smoothies, nut milks, and pâtés. But you can also use it to grind nuts, and chop vegetables—although a food processor might be more appropriate for that type of job. Basically you will use the Vita-Mix to turn foods into a liquid. As we do a lot of blending in the raw food cuisine, you will want something that totally blends, with almost no visible particles left. The Vita-Mix is suited for this.

CHAMPION JUICER—The Champion is another popular machine used in preparing raw foods. It is a mastication juicer that can juice soft fruits with ease, and is also used as a food processor. It can turn nuts into nut butters, or frozen fruit into ice cream. We use it to make all of our nut pâtés, and to make juice. It is fast and easy to clean. The downsides are that it cannot juice green vegetables very well, and tends to heat up the foods. Also, it cannot properly juice celery and other tough and fibrous vegetables.

GREEN POWER/GREEN LIFE JUICER—The Green Power Juicer is a step up from the Champion Juicer. It has been specifically designed to juice green vegetables. The Green Power Juicer uses twin gears, which crush the foods at a slow pace. It extracts the most out of fruits and vegetables, without heating them, thus preserving all of the enzymes and trace minerals. It also makes ice cream out of frozen fruits as well as nut butters just like the Champion. The downsides are that it is not the best juicer to juice fruits and it takes a little longer to clean. It remains our juicer of choice nonetheless. The Green Life juicer is very similar to the Green Power, made by the same company. It misses a few features, such as pasta making that you may not use anyway.

OTHER TYPES OF JUICERS—There are many types of juicers on the market that could be very useful in preparing raw foods. We will not discuss all of them in this book because we believe that the two juicers described earlier are the best investments one could make for the kitchen—and one's health.

DEHYDRATOR—The dehydrator is another popular tool used by many raw-foodists. With a dehydrator, you can dehydrate fruits and vegetables to preserve them, and also make delicious crackers, cookies, and other treats. The dehydrator could be considered the "oven" of the raw food cuisine.

It is important to use the dehydrator at a low heat so as to preserve the nutrients.

The dehydrator is an optional tool that is great to have, but not necessary. I realize that most people do not have a dehydrator. Because of this, I have separated out the few recipes in this book that need dehydration and placed them in a special section at the end of chapter 24. In case you are considering buying a dehydrator, the best brand on the market is the Excalibur dehydrator.

It comes with 4, 5, or 9 trays. I recommend getting either the 5 or 9 tray model, because they include a fan to regulate the temperature. If you buy a dehydrator, you will also need "Teflex" sheets, which are reusable plastic-like sheets that allow you to dehydrate wet/moist ingredients such as: crackers, crusts and other raw food recipes.

OTHER TOOLS USED

COFFEE GRINDER—The coffee grinder is used in the raw food cuisine to grind flax seeds, sesame seeds, and other seeds and small nuts. It's an inexpensive and useful tool to have.

FOOD PROCESSOR—Food processors still have their role in the kitchen, even if you already have the other tools described. Food processors are ideal for making crusts for living pies, for making date paste, and for grating cabbage and other vegetables.

SALADACCO—The Saladacco, also called the Spiralizer, is a little machine that we love. It turns vegetables like zucchinis, carrots, beets, and other hard vegetables into pasta-like strips. We use it to make garnishing for various dishes. It is a very fun tool that I think everyone should acquire.

CITRUS JUICER—Citrus juicers are usually inexpensive, and nice to have handy when making orange juice or other citrus juices. You can get a fairly good electric citrus juicer for less than $20.

Appendix 1

HOW TO TRANSITION TO A HEALTHY LIFESTYLE

Everyone is at a different stage in their dietary evolution. I wrote this book so that everyone, no matter where they are, can benefit from it. I do not condemn you if you still eat meat, dairy products, ice cream, sugar, and the other things that you know are less than excellent for your health. My job is not to make you feel guilty. Buying this book is proof that you are on your way to a better diet. Reading this book shows that you are interested in having more fruits and vegetables on your plate, less of the cooked and processed foods, and a more vibrant and healthy life.

A diet high in raw foods is a challenge for many people, and most, including myself, make the change to what I call the **"raw food lifestyle"** as a gradual process rather than as an overnight transformation. I will show you how you can ease into this lifestyle at a pace that is comfortable to you. I will also give you tips on how to cope with the difficulties you may encounter along the way.

First, understand that no matter what the state of your health is, you can benefit from eating more raw fruits and vegetables. Some people will feel that they are ready to eat all uncooked vegan foods, while others will gradually work their way into a healthier lifestyle. They will do this by eating more and more of the good foods, and less and less of the cooked and processed foods. We often hear about percentages to determine the level of commitment one has to a raw-vegan lifestyle. Some say, "I'm 80% raw," or "I eat 100% raw," meaning that 80% or 100% of what they eat is uncooked and unprocessed. These percentages reflect how far a person has decided to go with the raw food diet.

The first step to becoming a raw-vegan is obviously to eat more raw foods. Everyone should be eating at least 50% to 70% raw fruits and vegetables, no matter where they live, or what they do. Eating 50% to 70% raw fruits and vegetables is easier than you might think. As explained in the book **Fit for Life,** one should partake of fruits and/or juices in the morning. Because the body has been in an elimination period during the night, it is better not to stress the body with heavy food in the morning. So by eating healthy every morning, your body can continue the job of elimination that it was busy doing during the night.

It is good to start the day by drinking water I suggest drinking at least 10-20 ounces of water with some fresh lemon juice every morning. This will hydrate your body, and help flush out the toxins that have been eliminated from the cells during the night. It will also help the body to eliminate. Make sure that the water you drink is pure. Either purified, distilled, or a good-quality bottled water. When possible, get your water in glass bottles. Glass is cleaner, and does not carry any of the toxic components that plastic does. You can also get for about $30 a water purifier which will remove 98% of the toxic materials from tap water.

After you have your morning water, you may have some healthy beverages, such as freshly pressed juice. Have only liquids within the first two to three hours after waking. This will give your body a rest, and leave your mind clear and fresh.

Later in the morning, you may have some fruit if you feel hungry. Do not limit the quantity of fruit that you need to eat in order to satisfy your hunger. Eat as much as you want. You may eat two or three apples if you want. Most people are used to eating one apple once in a while. However, if you are to make a meal out of fruit only, you can eat more than one piece. Your taste buds will tell you when you have had enough of any one food.

For lunch, have a salad with avocado or some nuts. If you are eating cooked food, have only one kind and eat it with a salad. Always eat raw vegetables every time you eat cooked food. Have the salad first, and then have whatever else you want. If you must hve cooked food, have only one type, like a rice dish, some bread, or a soup. If you feel satisfied with your salad meal, why eat something else that would be less than excellent? Get on with your day. If you do not feel like having anything cooked for lunch, but do not feel totally satisfied with your salad, have something heavier. In addition to your salad, you could have guacamole, or other raw dips. Or maybe bring along a nut pâté, or simply some nuts and seeds to munch on. Also, olives can be very satisfying as a lunch-time snack.

During the rest of the day, eat fruit or raw vegetables when you feel like munching on something. Try to reduce your consumption of hot beverages, such as tea and coffee. Instead, drink more water. You may also try bringing a mix of nuts, seeds, and dried fruits as a snack to work.

For dinner, when you are home, make yourself a living soup and/or a salad. Experiment with some of the recipes in this book. You may accompany your meal with salad. If you feel like having an all raw meal, you could have guacamole, or nut pâté in a "burrito" (inside a lettuce or cabbage leaf).

If you still eat cooked food, but eat fruit in the morning, and a salad with every meal, plus have fruits and vegetables as snacks, you will be eating 50-70% raw, with almost no effort! Eating that way is both easy, and healthy. And you will enjoy it too. Prepare great dressings in advance and bring them along with you to work. When you make a recipe, make extra, and save some to bring with you to work. If you do not have time to prepare a meal in advance, then bring some raw fruits and vegetables along with nuts and seeds. Also, you can bring an avocado along with you, and eat it with a spoon, or add it to a salad at a restaurant. Many people bring their own salad dressings with them when they eat at restaurants.

Get in the habit of eating an abundance of raw fruits and vegetables. Eat lettuce and celery with everything. Bring carrot sticks with you in a plastic bag. Just get the raw food in! That is the first step. If you desire a beverage, make yourself a great juice in the morning. Apple-celery juice is a good choice. For dinner, start your meal with a green drink. Eat salad as a meal whenever possible. Experiment with fruits and vegetables you have never tried. Go to the market and get exotic fruits. Buy a new fruit or vegetable every week. Experiment with the variety Nature offers. Get your taste buds back into shape. Once you start eating more fruits and vegetables, they will become what you truly desire to eat. By filling your body with good nutrition, you will feel much better, and your body will request more.

After introducing better foods into your diet, you can start eliminating what is not healthy. The first type of food you want to avoid is processed food. Processed food is anything that comes in a can or from a factory, and contains additives and preservatives. It is also all the junk food that is served at the popular snack bars. So become health conscious, and refuse to eat refined sugar, refined flour, table salt, and foods that contain additives and/or preservatives. Stop shopping at the supermarket, and start shopping at the health food store. Buy organic food, and avoid anything that has been refined or processed in a food factory.

Other foods to be avoided are animal products and cooked starches. Animal products include fish, chicken, beef and pork, as well as dairy products such as milk, cheese, yogurt, and eggs. The consumption of animal products has been shown to be related to a variety of diseases, including cancer, heart disease, and diabetes. If you need a more in-depth explanation of what eating animals does to your health and the planet, I suggest reading the book, **Diet For A New America,** by John Robbins.

Many people in America are now becoming vegetarians for various reasons, health being one of them. It is known that, on average, vegetarians live longer than meat eaters, and experience fewer diseases. A vegetarian diet can do a lot for you, when it is practiced correctly. Vegetarians are becoming a part of the mainstream society, and most restaurants now carry vegetarian options. If none are listed, ask—they will frequently make one for you. Many people try to cut down on their meat intake, as they are learning about what a plant-based diet can do for them.

The downfall of the vegetarian diet is the high amount of cooked starches it often contains. Cooked starches include cooked grains and legumes, as well as the food items made from them such as bread, pasta, cookies, and crackers. It also includes baked potatoes. Most vegetarians eat a lot of these foods and, as a result, are not experiencing a high level of vitality. Many of the new diets in vogue these days, such as the Zone diet, promote fewer cooked starches (also called "carbohydrates"). Why? Because many people have found that eating cooked starches makes you gain weight, and may cause or aggravate many health conditions.

The trick to reducing, and eventually eliminating, the amount of starches you are eating is to eat starches no more than once or twice per day, and have only one type of starch at a meal. If you are going to have bread, then have bread, but not bread, potatoes, and rice. Also, there are some cooked starches that are easier on the body than others. Cooked sweet potatoes, or yams, for example, are a better choice than white potatoes. Brown rice is better than white rice. Sprouted bread is better than regular bread. Wheat products tend to be the worst type of cooked starch for many people. Wheat is a common allergen, and many find great relief in eliminating wheat products from their diet.

The last category of foods to reduce are all the other cooked and processed foods. This includes all the cooked vegetables, stewed fruits, and other cooked items. We have already discussed the issue of refined foods, so I am not going to talk here about all the condiments (ketchup, mustard, etc.), canned foods, and heavily processed and refined foods that you already avoid, and know to be bad for you. So that just leaves us with anything else that has been heated or processed.

Few people go as far as to eliminate all cooked foods from their diet, and for many it would seem an impossible goal that they would never be able to achieve. Many people would view such a move as quite radical and extreme. Yet, thousands of people throughout the world every year are learning about the benefits of eating raw plant foods, and deciding to let go of all cooked and processed foods. There will be a point in your dietary evolution where you will decide if you are ready to take this step. When this happens, just relax, let go, and embrace your new and fresh raw-vegan lifestyle. Nature will welcome you back into the world of pure and simple eating.

For those who are not ready to make such a move, or who feel it is not time for them, they can still benefit from increasing the amount of raw fruits and vegetables they are eating. They will still eat cooked foods, perhaps only on some occasions, but far less with every month that passes. For these people, we recommend cooked vegetables as the best choice of cooked food to eat. Starchless cooked vegetables, such as steamed kale, broccoli, spinach, zucchini, celery, cauliflower, peppers, and other vegetables, are quite healthy in comparison to cooked starches. Cooked or baked sweet potatoes (yams) are a more healthy food to eat than baked white potatoes.

When eating cooked foods, always eat a salad or other raw foods. If you bake a sweet potato, mash it in a bowl with some avocado, olive oil, and other seasonings. When eating steamed vegetables, top them with one of the salad dressings in this book or with any of the raw dips and raw sauces that you enjoy. Get the raw in with everything that you eat!

RAW FOODS IN THE WINTER

Another challenge that many people face when eating a raw-vegan diet is maintaining the lifestyle during the cold winters. Winter, for many of us, equals snow, cold, and a reduced variety of fresh fruits and vegetables available in the stores. Many people are used to drinking warm soups and other hot foods in the winter to stay warm, and feel that it would be hard for them to eat mainly raw foods during that time of the year.

First, it is good to know that eating hot foods will not necessarily make you warm. They will give you the illusion of being warm. Eating foods at room temperature will not necessarily make you feel cold, as long as you do not eat freezing foods, or fruit straight out of the fridge. The temperature of the food, in reality, has little effect on the ability of your body to produce internal heat. There are millions of animals living in the wild on Earth, eating only raw foods during the cold winter, and every one of them can handle the cold better than any of us so-called civilized humans. Would they be better off eating hot foods? I don't think so.

Meanwhile, we are not living with the animals in the wild, but in cities where things are quite different. Although our living conditions may be different than those of wild animals, our physiology is not. We are still bound by the same natural laws. As you improve your health with your diet, you should be able to withstand the cold much better, and will lose your desire for hot foods. It is possible that you might feel colder in the first months of your change of diet, as your body is adjusting and releasing toxins. But after a while, you will find that you can resist the cold much better.

In the winter time, I understand that warm foods such as soup may be comforting and enjoyable. If you would like to have a warm soup, here is a recipe that may help you:

Warm miso soup

2 cups **water**
2 Tbsp. **miso**
Small pinch of **sea salt** pinch of **cayenne pepper**
1 **garlic clove**
1/2 cup of your **favorite herb,** such as cilantro, parsley, or dill. (Optional)
2 Tbsp. **olive oil**

> Blend all ingredients except olive oil at high speed for a few seconds, and then pour into a pot. Warm up to desired temperature (keep under 110 degrees Fahrenheit). Add olive oil, mix well, and enjoy.

You can also warm up any of the soup recipes in this book, if you feel you want to have something hot. You do not have to cook them, but just warm them up.

It is much better to have something warm that is liquid, rather than a hot meal that is heavy. Liquid foods are always easier on the digestive organs.

Also, in order to go through the winter easier on a raw-vegan diet, there are a few other things you may want to try. One of them is to get some sunshine. I know that sun is scarce in the winter, but it is possible to get some sun on your skin. Exposure to even weak sun is great for your immune system, and enables you to go through the winter with more facility. The lack of sunshine during the winter causes many people to feel depressed. Some people have named this condition the "winter blues." To avoid this, get some sun on your skin regularly. You can stand naked behind a window when the sun shines through. Another way is to engage in outdoor activities. The sun tends to reflect greatly on the snow, and people often get sunburned while going skiing. You will benefit from limited exposure to the sun. Try to get the sun on your face, your hands, and as much of your body as you can safely and conveniently expose.

Exercise is a great way to fight the "SAD" winter blues (SAD: Seasonal Associated Depression/Seasonal Affective Disorder). There are many types of outdoor exercises that can be enjoyed during the winter, such as going for a brisk walk, or skiing. Don't get lazy because it is cold . . . keep going with your exercise program, and if you do not have one, think about starting one. If you can take time, go outside and play on the weekends. Also, keep exercising indoors by engaging in cardiovascular and resistance training.

Dr. Kristine Nolfi, who wrote **Raw Food Treatment of Cancer,** said that fruits and vegetables carry within them the sun's energy. She said that when a person eats a diet based on fruits and vegetables, they go through the winter without getting sick, and with much more ease and enjoyment. She was living in Denmark, where she had a successful retreat center treating people using raw fruits and vegetables. We should all listen to her advice, and understand how powerful these foods are for us. Many people eat a terrible diet during the winter, often eating foods that are totally devoid of life. Without the proper vitamins and nutrients, the immune system cannot function properly. Then these people get sick and wonder why. If they were to base their diet on fruits and vegetables, they would find that they would not get sick so often, even during the winter. They would go through the winter months with perfect enjoyment and ease.

By eating raw fruits and vegetables, exercising, and getting some sunshine, you will breeze through the winter with ease, and may even find yourself looking forward to the next winter. You can view winter as a time of cold, isolation, and boredom, or as a time of excitement, fun, and magic! Remember, how much you enjoy life has a lot to do with your selected perspective.

DETOXIFICATION PROCESS

As you improve your diet, it is inevitable that you will go through a healing process. Just like the smoker who stops smoking and proceeds to experience headaches and other discomforts, after you start following a cleaner diet, you go through what we call "detoxification." On a conventional diet, toxins accumulate in the body faster than they can be eliminated. The body, not being able to cope with all this toxic assault, stores these toxins in various places, with the intention to eliminate them later. When you improve your diet by eating less and by eating lighter foods, there is more body energy available. Digestion takes a lot of energy, and when you are eating heavy foods, such as bread and meat, a lot of this energy that your body has at its disposal is used to digest these heavy foods. When you eat a diet based on raw fruits and vegetables, you are freeing much of that burden, since these foods are easy to digest, and also due to the fact that you are bringing less toxins into the body.

Fruits and vegetables when eaten raw contain fewer toxins than cooked and processed foods. They also contain plenty of vitamins, minerals, and other nutritional components that your body can use to heal and maintain itself.

Someone said, "You have to feel worse before you can feel better!" This is often true. We cannot expect to eat junk food for decades, suddenly stop all of that, and then instantly feel better. Our bodies, when given the chance to heal and detoxify, will use that opportunity to get all of the garbage out.

To learn more about the process of detoxification, you should read my book **The Raw Secrets,** which goes into great detail on how to deal with conditions that may be experienced while the body is eliminating toxins. After you have improved your diet, remember to be easy with yourself. If you feel low one day, rest more and do something you enjoy. Keep your smile, and know that these discomforts are only temporary, and soon you will feel much better. Also, by spending more time outside and exercising, you will hasten the process of detoxification.

DEALING WITH FRIENDS AND FAMILY

When confronted with friends and family, a good attitude to have is to not try to convert everyone around you. Confronting someone about their diet is taboo, because people do not like to be told that what they are eating is unhealthy. They certainly do not want to be told what to eat. So do not try to convince anyone. Simply go on with your life. People who are interested in what you are doing will come to you. Then you can give them a book, and answer their questions. But, unless someone comes to you for guidance, there is no reason to try to convince anyone.

You do not have to talk about your diet. You do not have to tell anyone what you are doing. When you are invited somewhere, bring along your own food, and eat whatever healthy option they have for you. If they ask you questions, just say that you are on a special diet.

Remember, the idea here is to avoid confrontation. Do not engage in conversations about diet and food every time you visit friends and family. If you are in a more relaxed situation, with people who are open and understanding, you may then share some of your experiences. If you are not totally sure about the factual aspects of the vegetarian diet, just talk about your experiences with it. Talk about the benefits, without expecting them to believe every word.

In any case, do not fall into fanaticism. As you cannot be entirely sure that what you are doing is 100% right, there is no way you can know what is right for someone else. Do not think you have all the answers. Do not even think that your diet is "better." Simply follow what you think is best for your health, and if it doesn't seem to work for you, then try something else. We are all different so there is no way of eating that can work for everyone.

I have assumed in this chapter that you are already aware of the unhealthy but common substances such as: alcohol, tobacco, drugs, caffeine, and other obvious health-sappers. I have not discussed these topics, because I feel you are probably aware of these issues.

HERE'S TO YOUR RADIANT HEALTH

Your health is your most valuable asset, and you should care for it as well as you can. Invest in the best fuel to put in it, and treat your body like you would treat your most valuable possession. See your body as a temple, and with every mouthful of food that you put in it, see it as what you choose to bring to your temple.

Appendix 2
HYBRID FOOD AND WILD FOOD

Agriculture has been in existence for thousands of years, and throughout that time farmers have sought ways to improve their crops. Many techniques have been invented to modify the qualities of plants. For example, wild watermelons are quite bitter and not sweet. Wild almonds are poisonous. These foods have been hybridized using various methods, so now they are edible and pleasing to the taste. The various methods used in agriculture include selection, grafting, and crossbreeding. These methods have their benefits, since they have enabled us to eat many foods that we could not otherwise eat.

Hybridization is, after all, a natural process that many animals engage in. We eat fruits that we enjoy, and tend to propagate seeds of the plants that are the most pleasing to our taste. We then reproduce more of the plants that had pleasing qualities, such as sweetness. Farmers have done nothing more than copy what was actually done in Nature, by selecting the seeds that gave the best crops, and planting those seeds for the next season, instead of the seeds from the plants that gave poor results.

The downside of all this is that plants are now hybridized for reasons other than quality and taste. Nowadays plants are hybridized for commercial reasons such as to get bigger fruits, fruits with fewer "imperfections," cold-resistant plants, and plants that have less seeds, or other features that the markets request. We create plants that might have the physical qualities we seek, but have little taste and nutrition, to the point where most fruits and vegetables grown today by traditional methods, and often even organic methods, are incredibly tasteless, as well as low in vitamins and minerals.

Walk into your nearest supermarket, and you will see the lamentable reality. Shiny round apples with no taste, tomatoes without flavor, citrus that lacks sweetness, watery grapes with a detestable after-taste, and lettuce that has to be soaked in dressing to have any flavor at all. If our ancestors were still alive, they would likely express disappointment and disgust with today's produce, having been raised on foods that came from local gardens.

Many people, because of this, revert to the methods of our great-grandparents, and start to grow their own fruits and vegetables in their gardens. Not only do they enjoy the benefits of working outside in the soil, but they also enjoy the taste of food that is grown with love, not with dollar signs in mind. Gardening is the best solution to gaining access to good food.

Part of the reason many fruits and vegetables have no taste and little nutrition is that they are picked before maturity. When tomatoes are allowed to ripen on the vine, they have a totally different full-bodied taste than when they have been picked green and ripened using artificial methods. But the main reason why these fruits and vegetables are tasteless is that they have been grown from extremely hybridized seeds.

There were once over 7,000 varieties of apples. All of these were at one time grown in orchards throughout the world. Now you will be lucky to find more than five different varieties in your local supermarket. The varieties you will find are those that have been selected by the agribusiness to be the "best"—for economical reasons, not for taste or nutrition. They produce more, will ship without bruising, can withstand higher quantities of pesticides, and produce rounder fruits that the farmer thinks can be sold more easily.

Many people have grown up in a city, and have not had the experience of growing foods in a garden. Their way of selecting fruits and vegetables are those of the market, not those of experienced gardeners. They request fruits without imperfections, such as plastic-looking fruits. They do not realize that this is not the way real fruit appears in Nature. Fruits in Nature often acquire weird shapes, have imperfections, and do not resemble fruits found in most supermarkets. They are full of flavor and vitality. The shiny, round apples in your supermarket may look great as a decoration on your table, but are tasteless in comparison to natural apples.

People need to be educated about fruits and vegetables. They need to know how to select foods not simply according to their appearance, but according to their taste and nutritional quality. Once you start eating predominantly raw fruits and vegetables, this process becomes automatic. I can tell a good avocado in a basket of inferior ones just by the way they look. I can tell if it has been sitting on the tree long enough to have its full, buttery, fatty flavor. I know what a good avocado looks like because I have been buying avocados for years, and have lived where they grow. I know what a good mango looks like, as well as a good apple. I know that when I walk into my local supermarket there is little for me to eat because none of the fruit meets my criteria of quality.

Ancient varieties of fruits and vegetables have much more taste than the varieties grown today. Tomatoes from 100-year-old seeds have an amazing taste that is sweet and powerful—nothing like a commercial tomato, even one grown by organic methods. If you plan on getting the best food possible into your body, and you are considering the idea of growing some of your own food, I suggest that you get seeds of plants that have been less hybridized. You can find sources for these ancient seeds listed at the end of this book. *Seeds of Change* in New Mexico is an excellent source for quality heirloom seeds.

Many plants have been hybridized without limit, to the point where they cannot even reproduce themselves. Seedless fruits are an example of how the methods of hybridization have been taken to an extreme. Seedless fruits have been created because of the public's demand for fruits with fewer seeds. Even though it might be more convenient to eat seedless grapes than seeded grapes, the consequences are not worth that convenience. Foods that do not have seeds have a low life-force. They cannot reproduce themselves. They have been created to be commercial products in the big business of agriculture. They often tend to contain a type of sugar that is not handled well by the body. Bananas, for example, have a tendency to raise the blood sugar too fast. The sugar in apples, on the other hand, tends to be absorbed more slowly.

I suggest that you avoid all seedless fruits. If you are unable to grow your own, try to find and purchase grapes with seeds, and watermelon with seeds. Do not go with the trend and buy these seedless abominations. Fruit needs to have seeds. This is the way they naturally grow. Humans once ate fruit and propagated the seeds, thus reproducing the fruit trees everywhere. Now this natural circle has been broken, and it cannot be without consequences. Natural laws can never be broken without consequences.

A way to incorporate more nutritious food into your diet is to eat wild foods. Wild foods have never been tampered with by modern agricultural techniques, and contain their full nutrition and taste. For example, wild dandelion, a common weed that grows almost everywhere, contains more vitamins and minerals than the best commercial fruits and vegetables grown with the use of chemical fertilizers, and sometimes on rich soil. Wild dandelion contains more vitamin C, beta-carotene, and calcium than most fruits and vegetables sold in the store. And remember that the lowly dandelion grows without any watering, fertilizers, or other care. It often grows in very poor soil, and yet has such an amazing vitality, that it takes much human effort to get rid of it. We often say, "It grows like a weed," meaning that the plant grows everywhere without any human intervention. Farmers sure would like to see their plants grow like weeds! But no, they take care of their plants, water them, feed them, and with all of this, are never able to produce a plant that has anywhere close to the nutritional quality of a wild plant. Wild plants have such an amazing life-force and vitality because they have to fight for their lives in order to survive. They have to make the best use of what little they have.

Wild fruits and vegetables grow everywhere. There are some wild fruits and vegetables that grow where you are. All you have to do to find out which plants in your area are edible is to is pick up a copy of the book, **Guide to Edible Wild Plants of North America,** and go on a hike.

Asking the advice of a professional is also helpful. You can probably locate an herbalist in your area who will be happy to guide you on an edible wild plant tour.

Because of this understanding of wild foods versus hybridized foods, there are some foods that have been omitted from the recipes in this book, or used quite sparingly. Two categories of food that are not used in the raw food diet are grains and legumes. Grains are hybridized grass seeds. At the beginning, these seeds were not edible, and contained less starch. Through time, these seeds have been cultivated and hybridized to the point that they became starchier.

The hybridized grains used in mass-produced foods come from plants that have very little life-force. If you were to take a handful of wheat berries and throw them outside of the farmer's fence, and then return six months later, what would happen? Would anything grow from these seeds? Maybe. But they would likely be weak compared to their wild counterparts. These plants only seem to survive inside of the farmer's fence, with care and watering. They have little life-force, and due to their high starch content. The same thing holds true for legumes.

While it is not possible to revert entirely to wild foods, we can benefit from eating more wild foods, less hybridized foods, and by avoiding foods that are extremely hybridized, such as: grains, legumes, seedless fruits, and by growing our own food using ancient seeds.

Appendix 3

ORGANIC AND COMMERCIAL FOOD

Organic food is essential for health. I feel that it is not possible, in the long term, to maintain high levels of vitality while consuming commercially grown food. Go to the local supermarket and notice how the fruits and vegetables lack vitality. If you have ever taken care of a garden, you will realize how the fruits and vegetables available in the stores do not deserve their name. They are but pale shadows of their true potential. Shiny round apples without taste. Peppers and cucumbers covered with oil. Crisp lettuce that tastes like water. Mushy, genetically-engineered tomatoes. Disappointing melons. Watery avocados. And yet still more pale-looking, weak-tasting fruits and vegetables. All of these are sprayed heavily with pesticides, herbicides, and other toxic farming chemicals. Most likely they have been grown in soil filled with chemical fertilizers, and lacking in minerals. With the great advances of modern technology, chances are that one out of four fruits or vegetables found in your supermarket has been grown on plants that were genetically manipulated.

Organic foods contain more vitamins, minerals, and other nutrients than commercial foods. They also contain fewer toxic chemicals, since they are grown without the use of chemical fertilizers and pesticides.

Studies conducted in the United States by Dr. Victor Alexander, Director of Enviro-Health Systems, have shown that 99% of humans have pesticide residues in their blood. His research for this study was conducted on 3,000 people from around the world, and showed that 99% of them carried 4 types of pesticides in their blood on average. Sometimes as many as 19.

Pesticides are toxic to health. I do not have to spend time proving that fact. Each year, many people working on farms using pesticides die of the exposure to these toxic chemicals. The presence of pesticides in our bodies is quite alarming. Although it is generally admitted that pesticides are toxic, our health officials are trying to establish a tolerance level. They are indeed trying to figure out how much of these toxic chemicals we can ingest each year without suffering from immediate health problems. To create these standards, they take into account the reality of the average American, who is of an average weight, and who consumes an average quantity of fruits and vegetables.

The reality is that the optimum level of farming chemicals on your food should be "zero." While this is difficult, if not impossible, to accomplish, you can dramatically reduce the quantity of toxic substances you ingest by consuming organically grown produce. In addition, the current organic standards do not accept the use of genetically engineered seeds and food items.

MORE MINERALS IN ORGANIC FOOD

In addition to being free of most of the toxic chemicals that commercially grown food contains, organic food contains higher levels of minerals and trace minerals, which are extremely important for our health. According to research done in France, organic produce contained, on average, 26% more minerals than commercial produce, including 56% more calcium.

The fact is that organic farmers take better care of their soil. They try to put in the soil as much as they take out, in the form of good quality compost and natural fertilizers. Most commercial farmers, on the other hand, use harsh quick-grow chemical fertilizers that do not supply the soil with a wide range of all the trace minerals that we need. The goal of the typical chemically grown farm is to grow a lot of food as fast as possible, without much concern for its quality, in terms of its nutrition.

Organic food, while being more nutritious, also tastes better. You can taste the difference. When a friend of mine came to my house one day, and had one of my organic Canadian apples. He exclaimed, "Finally, an apple that tastes like something!"

Buying organic food is supporting your future. We vote with our dollars. This is real democracy. When you go to the store, and you purchase one thing instead of something else, you are voting. You are saying, "This is what I choose. This is the type of product I wish to see around." When you purchase organic food instead of commercial food, you are voting for a better future. You are supporting the farmers who are restoring the Earth, not the ones who are destroying it. You are saying, "This is what I want. I want organic food." As the demand grows, more farmers will be interested in becoming organic farmers. If no one purchases organic food because they think it is too expensive, then there is no demand, and many farmers will go out of business. If more people purchase organic food, then it will be easier for the distributors to sell at lower prices, as they get more bulk orders. On the other hand, when you are purchasing chemically-grown food, you are voting for an industry that is poisoning you and your children and destroying the land.

So remember that next time you go shopping. Is it really about the price? Do you really think that organic food is expensive? Is it worth it to save a few dollars, at the expense of ruining your health, the health of your children, and the future of life on this planet?

GENETICALLY-ENGINEERED FOODS

Walk inside your nearest supermarket. Do you notice much difference compared to 10 years ago? Besides the look and some new products, your supermarket probably does not seem any different than it was 10 years ago. You can probably find the same types of foods and products that were available there a decade ago. But, beyond all appearances, something major has changed. You do not recognize it because it is not mentioned anywhere. No labels will let you know that about two-thirds of all the products in your supermarket now contain ingredients that have been genetically-engineered. Two out of every three products in your supermarket have been tampered with in laboratories by scientists working for big biotech corporations.

If you live in North America, purchase your fruits and vegetables at the supermarket, and want to avoid genetically-engineered foods, all we can say is, "good luck." So far, 50 genetically-engineered (GE) crops have been approved by the U.S. Department of Agriculture, including potatoes, tomatoes, melons, and beets. GE rice, wheat, cucumbers, strawberries, apples, sugarcane, and walnuts are being grown on test sites. GE foods are everywhere, and are not allowed to be labeled as such by the government. It means that the government does not want you to be able to know the difference between a conventional tomato, and a genetically-engineered tomato. Why? Because they know that if consumers had the choice, they would not buy GE foods. They want to pass GE foods under your nose without you even knowing about it.

Genetically-engineered foods are foods that have been tampered with in laboratories at the genetic level. Genetic engineering creates entirely new types of plants by altering the genetic "blueprint" of these crops. By cutting, joining, and transferring genes between unrelated species, plants are created with unique qualities. Every plant or animal is unique because of the different genes contained within the cells of that organism. Genetic engineering is the process of modifying this information, and is light years beyond typical crossbreeding. As you already know, crossbreeding is a simple technique that has been used for thousands of years to alter crops and animals. It consists of interbreeding between two varieties of the same or similar species. Genetic engineering, though, is the Frankenstein version of this theme. In crossbreeding, farmers do not stray very far between species. Two vegetables of the same family could be crossbred together, but no one would ever have considered trying to crossbreed a tomato and a fish together Or would they? Now the barrier has been destroyed and it is possible to tamper with crops in such a radical way. The mutant tomato is a reality, and it is a quite a scary one.

For example, Edinburgh scientists have mixed jellyfish genes with potatoes, resulting in spuds that glow when they need watering. The idea was to plant a few of these per hectare for water monitoring purposes, and not for human consumption. We just wonder what will happen if the potatoes get mixed in with the regular batch.

Because genetic mistakes can never be recalled, GE poses one of the greatest dangers of any technology. Genetic defects are passed on to all subsequent generations, and their effect will spread out without limit.

One of the results of GE foods is that the technology may lead to the depletion of important food elements. Genetic engineers are capable of intentionally removing or inactivating a substance they consider undesirable in a food. The substance may have unknown but crucial qualities, such as cancer-inhibiting abilities.

GE foods that are tampered with to stay fresh longer might appear to be able to stay on the shelves for a longer period of time, but their nutritional content still decreases with every hour. And what would be the life-force of a food whose enzymes are so weak it cannot even ripen itself at a normal pace?

Since there is no labeling of GE foods, your only way to make sure that what you purchase has not been genetically engineered will be to purchase organic food exclusively, or grow your own food. Organic foods are not only more nutritious and free of the chemical fertilizers and pesticides that conventional foods contain, they are also certified to be non-genetically-engineered. They cost more than conventional foods, and might require a little effort to get, but in the end, understand that you pay now, or you pay later. There is just no other alternative.

EAT ORGANIC

Although the effect of pesticides are not felt immediately, it will not mean that they will not be felt in the long term. Many people feel that the dramatic increase in the occurrence of cancer in our society is an indication of the unforeseen damages of chemicals in our food. If you get cancer in 30 years, will you blame the commercial red bell peppers you ate all your life?

So the best insurance against this, as well as a support to the organic farming industry, is to eat as much organic food as possible starting today. When I say as much organic food as possible, I really mean: 100% by all means! Strive to eat 100% organic foods. If you cannot find organic peppers in February, well, why not just wait until next summer when they are in season again? Do you really want to eat those out-of-season peppers that have been imported from Mexico anyway, and possibly sprayed with toxic chemicals as third-world countries have less control over the amount of pesticides farmers are allowed to use? Avoid out-of season produce. This means eating cucumbers, tomatoes, and lettuce in the summer, not in the winter. It also means eating apples in January, not the ones imported from New Zealand in July. Eating what is locally in season is also in harmony with Nature, as it is the way we are supposed to eat.

All big cities have health food stores that carry organic produce. If you have to drive an hour or so to get there, because you are living outside of the city, well, that is what you will have to do. Understand that there are not many alternatives to organic. The supermarket is not an alternative. Growing your own food is though. You can have a garden, or even grow sprouts and greens indoors. Then you get the best foods ever, 100% organic, certified by yourself!

MOST HEAVILY SPRAYED CROPS

I understand though that sometimes you will be caught somewhere with no organic food around. It happens to me sometimes. So here is a list that could be helpful.

The following crops have been found to hold high amounts of toxic residues. The research that I used is taken from the book **Diet for a Poisoned Planet** by David Steinman. Research has studied only the part of the fruits that are eaten. For example, when analyzing a cantaloupe, researchers took into consideration only the flesh of the fruit.

High-Pesticide Residue Fruits and Vegetables (in North America) include: strawberries, cantaloupes (from Mexico), apples, pears, spinach, raisins, grapes, peppers, cucumbers, peanuts, celery.

The following crops are relatively safe. They are our choices when organically grown foods are not available. Remember that this does not guarantee that they will not be genetically-engineered, but at the year of publication (2001), these foods should not be. Remember that most of these items still contained pesticide residues, but in much smaller quantities than in the other foods analyzed.

Relatively Safe Fruits & Vegetables (in North America) include: papayas, watermelons, citrus (except tangerines), corn, cabbage, all nuts except peanuts.

A last point: some people complain that organic food is too expensive and that they cannot afford it, since they have a low income and a large family to feed. My answer is that you either pay now, or you will pay later. Look at it this way: how much will it cost when you and your children suffer from the long-term effects of pesticide poisoning? With the introduction of these genetically-engineered foods, how much will it cost you to face the now-unknown long-term effects resulting from the consumption of such foods? How much is that worth? Is that worth the price? Do you really save anything in the end when you are encouraging an industry that destroys our precious planet?

We have to realize that as more people start eating organic foods, it will become more affordable and more available. The organic food industry is a blossoming industry currently growing at the rate of 20% per year. It is very exciting to be part of a movement that is working toward bringing back real food onto our tables.

As a last word to conclude this work. I would like to thank all of you who invested money to buy this book, and invested your time to learn to eat better.

I hope you had as much fun reading this book as I had writing it, and that by now you understand the basic concept behind it: *to be alive, eat alive.*

BIBLIOGRAPHY

Alexander, Joe, **Blatant Raw-Foodist Propaganda,** (Blue Dolphin, 1990).

Arlin, Dini, Wolfe, **Nature's First Law: the Raw-Food Diet** (Maul Bros., 1999).

Arlin, Stephen, **Raw Power,** (Maul Bros., 1998).

Burger, Guy Claude, **Instinctothérapie: Manger Vrai** (Édition du Rocher, 1990).

Cousens, Dr. Gabriel, **Conscious Eating** (North Atlantic Books, 2nd Edition).

Diamond, Harvey & Marilyn, **Fit For Life,** (Mass Market Paperback, 1987).

Esser, William L, **Dictionary of Natural Foods,** (Natural Hygiene Press, 1983).

Gagnon, Yves, **La culture écologique** (Éditions Colloïdales, 1984).

Howell, Dr. Edward, **Enzyme Nutrition: the Food Enzymes Concept,** (Avery Publishing Group, 1986).

Kulvinskas, Viktoras, **Survival into the 21st Century,** (21st Century Publication, 1993).

Marcus, Erik, **Vegan: the New Ethics of Eating,** (Mc Books Press, 1998).

Meyerowitz, Steve, **Sprouts: the Miracle Food,** (Sproutman Publications, 1999).

Onstad, Dianne, **Whole Foods Companion,** (Chelsea Green, 1996).

Safron, Jeremy; Underkoffer, Renée, **The Raw Truth: the Art of Loving Foods** (Raw Truth Press, 1997).

Shelton, Herbet, **Food Combining Made Easy** (Willow Publishing, 1940).

Steinman, David, **Diet for a Poisoned Planet,** (Harmony Books, 1990).

Wigmore, Ann, **The Sprouting Book,** (Avery Publishing Group, 1986).

Wolfe, David, **The Sunfood Diet Success System,** (Maul Bros., 2000).

Wolfe, David, **Eating For Beauty,** (Maul Bros. 2002).

Contact the Author

For any other queries or comments on this book,
you can e-mail the author by sending in a support ticket at:.

Email: fredericpatenaudesupport.com

To keep in touch with what is going on in the raw-vegan
world, please visit the following website regularly:

http://www.rawforlife.net